Minimally Invasive Urologic Surgery

Minimally Invasive Urologic Surgery

A Step-by-Step Guide

Qais Hooti, MD, SB-Urol

Consultant Urologist, The Royal Hospital, Muscat, Oman
Member of Oman Urology Society
Member of Oman Medical Specialty Board

Sung-Hoo Hong, MD, PhD

Professor, Department of Urology and Director of Urologic Cancer Centre,
Seoul St. Mary's Hospital, The Catholic University of Korea
Director of Robot Surgery Committee, Korean Urological Association
Director, Korean Renal Cancer Study Group
Director of Education Committee, Korean Urological Oncology Society
Member of Board of Directors, Korean Endourological Society
Member, American Urological Association
Member, Endourological Society
Member, Societe Internationale d'Urologie

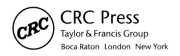

CRC Press
Taylor & Francis Group
Boca Raton London New York

CRC Press is an imprint of the
Taylor & Francis Group, an **informa** business

First edition published 2023
by CRC Press
6000 Broken Sound Parkway NW, Suite 300, Boca Raton, FL 33487-2742

and by CRC Press
4 Park Square, Milton Park, Abingdon, Oxon, OX14 4RN

CRC Press is an imprint of Taylor & Francis Group, LLC

© 2023 Taylor & Francis Group, LLC

Library of Congress Cataloging-in-Publication Data
Names: Hooti, Qais, author. | Hong, Sung-Hoo, author.
Title: Minimally invasive urologic surgery : a step-by-step guide / Dr Qais Hooti, Dr Sung-Hoo Hong.
Description: First edition. | Boca Raton : CRC Press, 2022. | Includes bibliographical references and index. |
Summary: "This text provides concise and highly practical information covering the most commonly performed urological procedures. Each procedure is presented in detail, supported by scientific justification and supplemented by operative images and diagrams. The operative steps are clearly explained with critical moments highlighted. The content is organized to enable the reader to both understand and identify the key teaching points and tricks to achieve optimal results. * Focuses on the technical aspects of surgery to ensure improved surgical technique * Easy to read, understand and apply the information * Enhanced by tips and tricks to provide further insights into clinical practice. Of great value and assistance in surgical laparoscopy and Robotic surgery courses, and in urology residency training and fellowship programs"—Provided by publisher.
Identifiers: LCCN 2021062729 | ISBN 9781032257105 (paperback) | ISBN 9781032257143 (hardback) | ISBN 9781003284666 (ebook)
Subjects: MESH: Nephrectomy | Prostatectomy | Laparoscopy—methods |
Robotic Surgical Procedures—methods | Urologic Diseases—surgery | Handbook
Classification: LCC RD571 | NLM WJ 39 | DDC 617.4/610597—dc23/eng/20220204
LC record available at https://lccn.loc.gov/2021062729

ISBN: 9781032257143 (hbk)
ISBN: 9781032257105 (pbk)
ISBN: 9781003284666 (ebk)

DOI: 10.1201/b22928

Typeset in Galliard Std
by codeMantra

I dedicate this work to my mother, my wife and my daughters, without whom my success would have never been possible

Qais Hooti

If you want to make surgery easy, expose it well

Use natural traction by gravity

Do not count the number of trocars

It is not a shame to convert to open surgery

If you want to have surgery fast, slow it down

Sung-Hoo Hong

Contents

Preface...ix
Acknowledgments...xi

SECTION 1 **BASIC INSTRUMENTATION** 1

CHAPTER 1
Patient Positioning, Operating Room Setup and Surgeon's Posture................................... 3

CHAPTER 2
Instruments and Machines.. 7

CHAPTER 3
Entry and Exit.. 19

SECTION 2 **LAPAROSCOPIC UROLOGIC SURGERY** 27

CHAPTER 4
Transperitoneal Laparoscopic Radical Prostatectomy 29

CHAPTER 5
Transperitoneal Laparoscopic Radical Nephrectomy 51

CHAPTER 6
Transperitoneal Laparoscopic Radical Nephroureterectomy 69

CHAPTER 7
Transperitoneal Laparoscopic Partial Nephrectomy 89

CHAPTER 8
Retroperitoneal Laparoscopic Simple Nephrectomy 109

CHAPTER 9
Laparoscopic Radical Cystoprostatectomy.. 119

CHAPTER 10
Extracorporeal Urinary Diversion (Modified Studer Orthotopic Ileal Neobladder) and Intracorporeal Urethra-Neobladder Anastomosis...**137**

SECTION 3   **ROBOT-ASSISTED UROLOGIC SURGERY** **147**

CHAPTER 11
Transperitoneal Robot-Assisted Laparoscopic Radical Prostatectomy **149**

CHAPTER 12
Transperitoneal Robot-Assisted Laparoscopic Partial Nephrectomy **169**

CHAPTER 13
Retroperitoneal Robot-Assisted Laparoscopic Partial Nephrectomy **187**

Bibliography 201
Index 207

Contents

Preface

Performing a surgical procedure is of great value when it is accompanied by a comprehensive understanding of its underlying science. The ability of reasoning and explaining each surgical step and its clinical application differentiates a surgeon from an operator.

Minimally invasive surgery is considered the standard of care for various abdominal urological pathologies and therefore requires state-of-the-art surgical skills. Transferring knowledge through well-written and illustrated manuals and atlases is crucial to understanding the operative steps and improving technical abilities. Several authors have used different strategies of writing to deliver their information to the reader in as easy, interesting, attractive and practical method possible.

This manual is the fruit of the collective experience during fellowship training with high-volume surgeons at Seoul St. Mary's Hospital (The Catholic University of Korea) in South Korea. During fellowship, the curiosity to learn every minute operative detail peaks to gain the maximum level of surgical quality of skills and understanding.

This step-by-step guide to minimally invasive urologic surgery is a concise and highly practical notes style book focusing on the most commonly performed urological procedures. Each procedure is presented in detail, supported by scientific justification and reasoning and supplemented by real operative images and diagrams. The operative steps are clearly explained and the critical moments are distinctly highlighted. It is organized to serve the reader for better understanding and easier identification of the key teaching points and tricks to achieve optimal results.

The main purpose of writing this book is to enable young urologists to reproduce and master the techniques and successfully overcome operative challenges.

Acknowledgments

Deepest gratitude is to our families and friends who always support and motivate us. We are extremely grateful to our surgical assistants Seung Chol Han, Goon Ho Kang and Hyeoksam Kwon for their endless efforts and collaboration. We also extend our appreciation to the urology residents, fellows and professors for their invaluable contribution and advice. Sincere thanks to the operating room nurses who were always ready to assist and provide the necessary materials.

Qais Hooti
Sung-Hoo Hong

Basic Instrumentation

Patient Positioning, Operating Room Setup and Surgeon's Posture

1

- Appropriate and specific operating room setup with patient positioning and surgical team location for each procedure is essential to facilitate the flow of the surgery.
- The optimal patient position differs depending on the procedure performed, aiming for easy access and accurate handling of instruments.
- Establishing a safe patient position is the responsibility of surgical team members.
- Malpositioning is associated with considerable patient morbidities and surgical complications.
- To prevent position-related injury events, the patient has to be carefully supported by gel pads, sand bags, adhesive tapes and belts, and the pressure points have to be well secured (Figure 1.1).

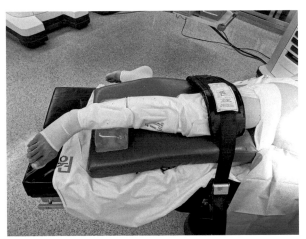

Figure 1.1 Patient is stabilized by adhesive tape and belt. The cautery pad, elastic stocking and pneumatic compression devices are applied. The pressure areas are supported by the gel pad.

- Elastic stockings and/or intermittent pneumatic compression device are applied and connected.
- All tubes and cable connections must be carefully placed, fixed and secured.
- The lines should not obscure the field, or interfere with the surgeon's arm movements or instrument handling.
- Accessory machines such as the insufflator and hemostasis generator are preferably placed within the surgeon's visual field.
- The physical or posture ergonomics in laparoscopy are more challenging in comparison to robotic surgeries.
- Incorrect patient positioning or surgeon posture will negatively affect task performance, quality of work and may lead to increased risk of technical errors and complications.
- Incorrect patient positioning or surgeon posture causes stress and fatigue to the surgeon, in addition to musculoskeletal pain and inflammation such as cervical spondylitis and tenosynovitis.

DOI: 10.1201/b22928-2

- The operation table height is adjusted in relation to the arms so the instrument handle are slightly below the surgeon's elbow.
- The best working angle at the elbow joint should be between 90° and 120° and the arms should be just abducted (Figure 1.2).

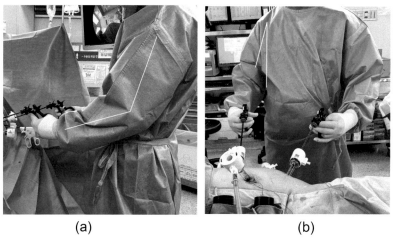

(a)   (b)

Figure 1.2 Working angles. (a) At the elbow joint. (b) At the shoulder joint.

- This necessitates the table to be as low as 49% of the surgeon's height, which equals to an average of 70 cm from the floor.
- The distance between the working instruments should not be very wide requiring increased shoulder abduction, which may cause fatigue or handling difficulties.
- To achieve the correct posture, it may be necessary to step up on a stand or a stool, taking care of possible fall and injuries.
- The surgeon's position should be aligned with the scope, target organ and the monitor (coaxial alignment) (Figure 1.3).

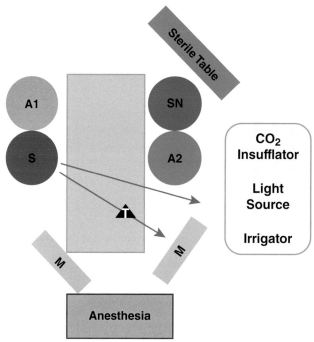

Figure 1.3 Diagram showing the operating room setup. Note the coaxial alignment of the surgeon (S) position, target organ (T) and monitor (M). The accessory machines are in the surgeon's visual field.

- The monitor height is set at 25° from the horizontal plane of the surgeon's eyes; so, prolonged neck extension and muscular spasm are avoided (Figure 1.4).

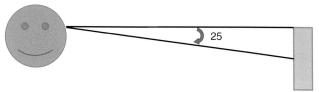

Figure 1.4 Diagram showing the height of the monitor, which is set at 25° below the horizontal plane of the surgeon's eyes.

- The distance between the surgeon and the monitor must be adequate depending on the screen size.
- A far or close distance will strain the eyes and negatively affect the clarity of the image.

2 Instruments and Machines

THE DA VINCI XI ROBOTIC CART

- The patient cart should be checked and prepared before starting each procedure.
- The arms are draped by the scrub nurse using the sterile plastic drape and kept in a safe area to avoid contamination by operation room members.
- Once the patient is in final position and all robotic trocars are inserted, the circulating nurse will drive the robotic cart to the correct side and location in relation to the patient.
- The patient's side surgeon (assistant) should guide the circulating nurse to guide the cart to the accurate position to the patient body using the green laser mark.

INSUFFLATOR

- The insufflator is preferably located in the surgeon's visual field to monitor pressure and gas flow during access and throughout the procedure.
- The adequacy of gas should be checked before each surgical session or early in the day.
- CO_2 flow is set at a low rate until the correct position of the Veress needle is confirmed.

Confirmation of correct Veress needle passage and position is explained in Chapter 3, Section 1 "Basic Instrumentation".

- The pressure is set to at least 15 mmHg during trocar insertion and then it is decreased to 12 mmHg throughout the procedure.
- Increasing the intraperitoneal pressure to 20 mmHg for a short period (10 minutes) may occasionally be required if significant bleeding is anticipated, e.g., during deep vascular complex transection in robotic prostatectomy.

ENERGY DEVICES AND HEMOSTATIC GENERATORS

- The electrocautery or ultrasonic machines are set according to the approach (laparoscopic or robotic) and the type of instrument being used.
- High-energy ultrasonic shear (Harmonic Scalpel from Ethicon or Thunderbeat from Olympus) is the authors' preferred dissector for laparoscopic procedures.

The blade of the ultrasonic shear becomes very hot once activated, so it is mandatory to avoid blade contact to vessels or intestinal surfaces, after activation.

- The ultrasonic instrument is prepared, connected and tested by the scrub nurse at the beginning of the procedure.
- If electrocautery is used, the grounding pad should be well placed and the foot paddle is located at the surgeon's side.

DOI: 10.1201/b22928-3

CAMERA (LAPAROSCOPE)

- Scopes of size 8 and 10 mm are used for da Vinci Xi robot and laparoscopic procedures, respectively, with 0° and 30° lens depending on the type of surgery.
- In laparoscopic surgeries, the 30° scopes are usually challenging to the inexperienced assistant, especially in the early stages of training.
- The view can easily disorient the surgeon to the anatomy, leading to unwanted events or errors.

ULTRASOUND PROBE

- An endoscopic 10-mm ultrasound probe can be utilized in partial nephrectomy procedures to localize the tumor and assess its margins in order to decide the width and depth of dissection.
- It may also be used in assessing the kidney vascularity and extension of inferior vena cava (IVC) thrombus in cases of radical nephrectomy and IVC thrombectomy.

SCRUB NURSE SURGICAL TABLE

- In addition to the laparoscopic instruments, the surgical sterile table should also include the open surgery set, which must be readily available in case of emergency conversion.
- The laparoscopic instruments include Veress needle, trocars, retractors, balloon dilator, scissors, graspers, dissectors, clip appliers, staplers, vascular clamps, suction probe, hemostatic agents, Carter Thomason device and entrapment endo-catch bag.
- In addition, other material supplies such as marking pens, ruler, vessel loops, gauze, skin retractors, syringes and suture materials should be available.
- **Maryland grasper** is used as a dissector, retractor and for retrieval of small specimens or biopsies in addition to the introduction and removal of supplies such as gauze pieces and sutures.
- **Right-angled dissector** is used to dissect the tissues and blood vessels particularly for creating planes and windows before clipping, stapling or transecting them.
- The instrument handling technique may differ according to the surgeon's preference and the task being performed (Figure 2.1).

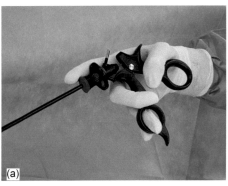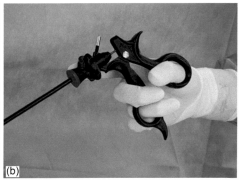

Figure 2.1 Handling the instrument. (a) Simple dissection for long time. (b) Fine dissection for short time.

- Prolonged improper handling may lead to numbness, hand muscle pain or sensory nerve injury of the thumb.
- **Babcock forceps** is used to gently grasp and retract the tissue or organs without causing vascular damage or tissue injuries, e.g., the ureter during mobilization at cystectomy surgery (Figure 2.2).
- **Atraumatic locking grasper** is used for retracting the liver and grasping structures such as vas deference and ureter to provide wide exposure during dissection (Figure 2.3).

SUCTION-IRRIGATION

- The suction-irrigation functions must be checked before starting the procedure.
- Ensuring that the trocar skin site allows the suction probe tip to reach the target area is essential.
- A 5-mm probe is used to irrigate the fluid and clear the field of smoke and blood (Figure 2.4).

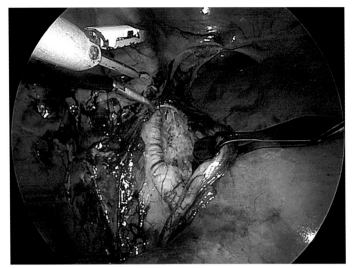

Figure 2.2 Using Babcock forceps for non-traumatic retraction of the left ureter during radical cystectomy.

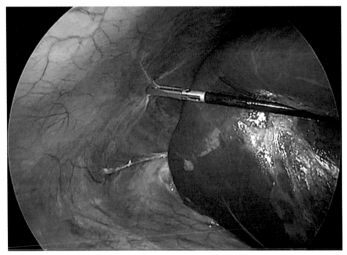

Figure 2.3 Atraumatic locking grasper retracting the liver.

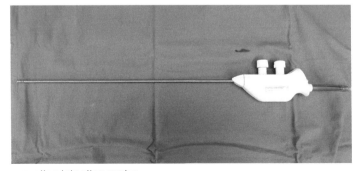

Figure 2.4 A 5-mm suction-irrigation probe.

- The suction-irrigation probe may also be used as blunt dissector by the surgeon or as a retractor by the assistant when there is no bleeding requiring suction.
- The usual irrigant is normal saline and may need to be delivered under pressure using automatic pump like Endomat from Storz.

RETRACTORS

- The S-shape retractors are used for fascial layer exposure during open access approach (Figure 2.5).

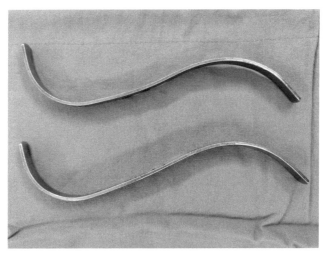

Figure 2.5 S retractors.

- A laparoscopic 10-mm fan retractor with safe, blunt, malleable ends provides a wide area of retraction (Figure 2.6).
- The suction probe and graspers may be used for the same purpose.

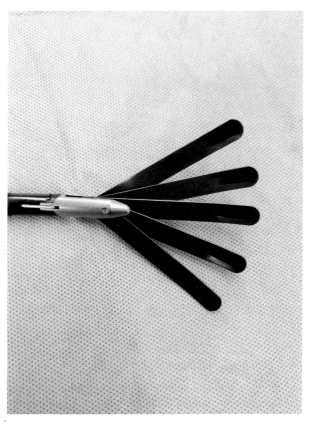

Figure 2.6 Fan retractor.

SUTURES

- Suture materials and size of needles used differ according to the purpose and task being performed.
- V-Loc stitch is the suture material of choice for kidney reconstruction, vesicourethral anastomosis, bladder cuff cystostomy closure and neobladder formation.
- PDS is utilized for deep vascular complex ligation, second layer renorrhaphy and as retraction stitch to the abdominal wall.
- Vicryl and silk suture materials are used for wound closure and fixation of the drain to the skin, respectively.

NEEDLE DRIVERS

- Left- and right-hand needle drivers are available for comfortable handling and accurate suturing (Figure 2.7).
- The needle driver with curved jaws that allows the surgeon to change the needle direction is preferred.

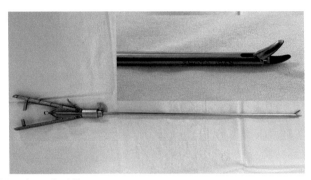

Figure 2.7 Needle driver from Karl Storz.

SUTURING MANEUVER

- For laparoscopy suturing, the stitch is introduced through the port using the right-hand needle driver by holding the thread 1–2 cm from the needle.
- The needle is then grasped by the left hand, and to achieve optimal orientation, it may need to be rotated and adjusted by manipulating the thread using the right hand.
- The needle is held at the correct side of the jaws (curved one), perpendicular to its axis at the 2/3–1/3 parts.
- Occasionally, the needle may need to be held at a certain angle to achieve a precise suturing at the tissue level.

> For precise and easy suturing in laparoscopy, it is essential to have an optimal manipulation angle of around 60° between the instruments (Figure 2.8).

- To achieve an optimal suturing angle, it may occasionally be necessary to stabilize the organ by another instrument or by a traction stitch using a suture passer needle (Figure 2.9).
- The needle should be introduced perpendicular into the tissue and advanced with rotational movement (supination or pronation).

To avoid laceration injuries, the needle must be removed at the tissue exit by rotational movement with its curve.

> The needle exit point is more important than the entry one, therefore when driving the needle through the tissue it must be directed to the desired exit.

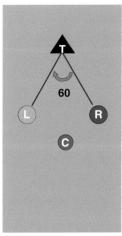

Figure 2.8 Diagram showing the optimal manipulation angle (60°) between the instruments during suturing. *Abbreviations*: C, camera; T, target organ; R and L, right and left ports.

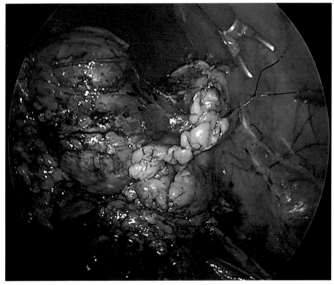

Figure 2.9 Kidney stabilization by a stitch during partial nephrectomy to achieve optimal suturing angle.

Pulling the stitch tightly by holding the needle may cause intra-abdominal injuries or can cut off the thread from the needle.

- The needle is preferably removed out of the body through the port using a needle holder by grasping the thread rather than the needle itself.
- In case the thread is too short to be grasped, then it is preferred to straighten the needle if possible with caution using robotic or laparoscopic needle drivers, so it can be grasped and removed safely.

BULLDOG VASCULAR CLAMPS

- Bulldog vascular clamps are used in partial nephrectomy and IVC thrombectomy to clamp the major vessels, during resection and suturing (Figure 2.10).
- Using the Bulldog clamp applicator and remover for precise control at the level of the vessels is crucial.
- If both the renal artery and vein need to be clamped during partial nephrectomy, two Bulldog clamps may be used separately. Alternatively, a laparoscopic Satinsky clamp can be utilized to control both vessels together.

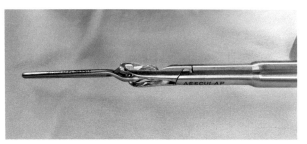

Figure 2.10 Bulldog vascular clamp and the applicator.

SCISSORS

- Laparoscopic scissors can be straight or curved.
- Straight scissors are used for cutting stitches or dividing the structure in-between closely placed clips.
- Curved scissors are used for dissection and can be attached to electrocautery diathermy.

CLIPS AND CLIP APPLICATORS

- Two types of clips are used, the nonabsorbable polymer plastic locking clips (Hem-o-lok) and titanium clips (Ligaclip) (Figure 2.11).

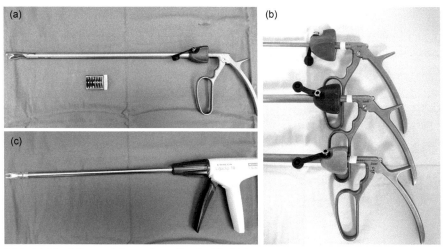

Figure 2.11 (a) Size L Hem-o-lok applier with clip kit. (b) Hem-o-lok clip appliers, different colors point to different sizes. (c) Titanium ligaclip applier.

- The clips are different sizes depending on the structure or tissue volume/diameter to be clipped.
- They can already be preloaded in the applier or to be loaded manually depending on the type used.
- The tips of the clip appliers can be straight at 0° or angular at 20° or 45°.
- Tissue dissection and/or window creation particularly for large vessels is performed before clipping.
- The clip is advanced maximum on the structure aiming to encapsulate it completely.
- The Hem-o-lok applier is gently rotated so the single tooth at the tip of the clip is seen from the other side of the structure.
- The clip tips are approximated (but not locked), and slid maximum to one side of the structure to provide a safe distance for the other clip before division (Figure 2.12).

For accurate and safe clip ligation of a large vein, surrounding it by a vessel loop allows for a gentle traction to open a window around the vein and will shrink or decrease the circumference of its wall.

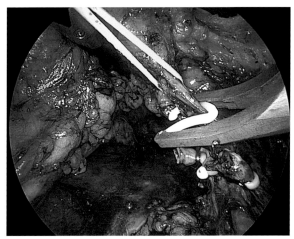

Figure 2.12 Clipping technique of renal vein using a vessel loop to shrink its wall. The end teeth of the clip are approximated before sliding it to one end of the vein. Note the angle orientation of the applicator.

- Locking mechanism should be performed in a careful manner, especially during clipping a major vessel, so that no tissue or vessel wall is entrapped between the end teeth.
- The force applied on the applier handle should be sufficient enough to close the clip.
- The applier is removed slowly and carefully making sure the jaws are well opened and not stuck to the clip or the tissue.
- A 3-mm distance from the clip is provided as a safety margin before division, and clipping on a clip must be avoided.

> To provide a wider space between the clips for safe transection, particularly in short structures, the angular curves of clip applier tips are directed away from the intended line of division (Figure 2.13).

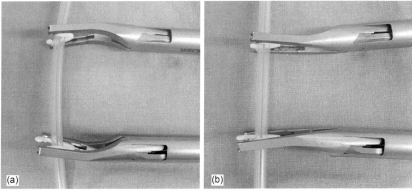

(a) (b)

Figure 2.13 Clipping technique. (a) Wide space between the clips. (b) Short space.

STAPLERS

- For bowel resection and anastomosis, during neobladder formation, a 60 mm × 3.8 mm GIA stapler (DST series) from Covidien is used (Figure 2.14a).
- A 12-mm diameter GIA with a 60 mm × 2.5 mm cartridge stapler is used for controlling the bladder pedicle in radical cystectomy.
- Endoscopic GIA (Endo-GIA Ultra, Universal Stapler from Covidien) can articulate and deflect at the tip, allowing a greater range of angles for accurate application (Figure 2.14b and c).

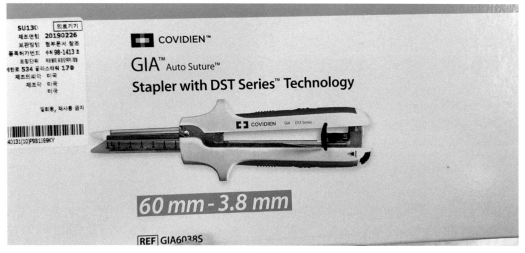

(a)

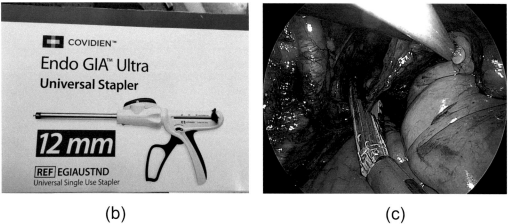

(b)   (c)

Figure 2.14 GIA staplers: (a) for bowel resection anastomosis, (b) articulating Endo-GIA ultra and (c) articulation during bladder pedicle control.

It is important to ensure absence of any clips at the area being stapled to prevent misfiring or malfunctioning of the device.

HEMOSTATIC AGENTS

- Hemostatic agents are utilized in the bleeding areas, which are not amenable for cauterization, clip application or suture ligation.
- Different products are available, but those used for this manual's procedures are Surgicel, TachoSil and FloSeal.
- Surgicel is made of oxidized *cellulose* polymer and manufactured by *Ethicon*.
  - It is absorbable and can be cut to small sizes appropriate to cover the bleeding area.
- TachoSil is made of *collagen* and coated with *fibrinogen* and *thrombin*.
- The TachoSil sponge is made from horse tendons and its active side is colored in yellow.
  - It can be cut to smaller sizes or be rolled (bolster) as for renorrhaphy in partial nephrectomy procedures (Figure 2.15).
- FloSeal is a hemostatic matrix of gelatin granules and thrombin.
  - It comes in a pack of 5 mL to be mixed and prepared by the scrub nurse during surgery and is applied on the dissection area, e.g., prostate bed for at least 5 minutes.

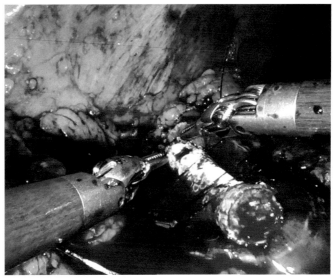

Figure 2.15 A hemostatic agent TachoSil (bolster) in renorrhaphy during partial nephrectomy.

SPECIMEN RETRIEVAL

- The small tissue sampling or biopsy can be removed by using a Maryland grasper.
- Small specimens such as lymph nodes in pelvic lymphadenectomy can be retrieved using a gloved finger.
- For larger specimens, an endo-catch bag is used, and appropriate size should be selected to fit the resected mass (Figure 2.16).
  - The bag is closed by pulling the thread through the port and the thread is clipped by Hem-o-lok to ensure the closure.

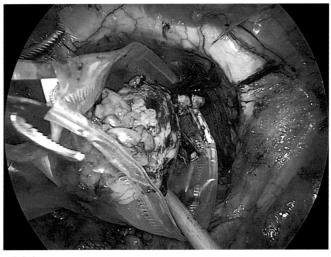

Figure 2.16 Endo-catch bag.

DRAINS

- The Jackson-Pratt drain is the authors' preference for the performed procedures; however, other drain types can be efficiently used (Figure 2.17).

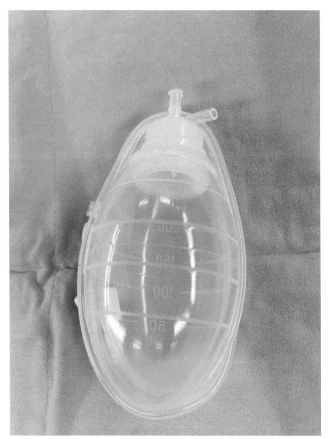

Figure 2.17 Jackson-Pratt drain.

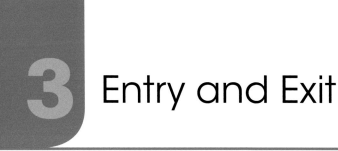

3 Entry and Exit

ACCESS

- The transperitoneal laparoscopic access can be achieved by a closed method (using Veress needle) or by an open (Hasson) technique.
  - Before inserting the Veress needle, it is important to ensure the spring (retraction) mechanism is working and the lumen is not obstructed allowing free flow of saline.
- The urinary bladder is emptied by a Foley catheter and a nasogastric tube may be required.
- The abdominal wall around the needle entrance point is grasped by towel clips and stabilized.
- The Veress needle is held like a dart and inserted perpendicular to the abdominal wall of the patient (Figure 3.1).

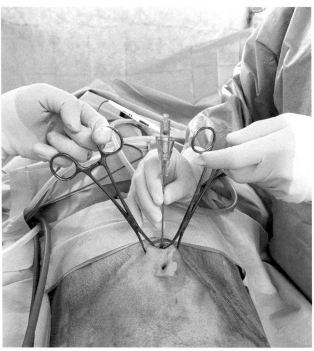

Figure 3.1 Insertion of the Veress needle perpendicular to the abdominal wall, which is stabilized by two towel clips. Note the needle is held like a dart.

DOI: 10.1201/b22928-4

- The correct position of the Veress needle in the abdominal cavity must be confirmed before starting CO_2 insufflation (Figure 3.2).

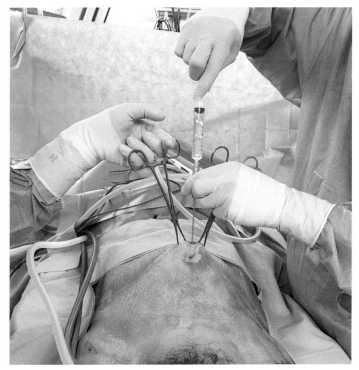

Figure 3.2 Water test of Veress needle tip position.

Confirmation of Veress needle correct passage and position:

1. Two click sounds: sensation of giving way passing through
   First: the rectus fascia.
   Second: the transversalis fascia and peritoneum.
2. Aspiration: few bubbles, no blood, urine or fecal contents.
3. Saline (injection) irrigation: free flow without resistance.
4. Aspiration (recovery): no fluid should be recovered back.
5. Hanging drop test: a saline drop is sucked into the abdomen.
6. Low intra-abdominal pressure (<7 mmHg) with low gas flow.

- For open (Hasson) technique, around 2-cm skin incision is made at the intended port site, and the wound is opened in layers by fascial cutting and muscle splitting using a straight hemostat.
- An optimal wound exposure can be achieved by S retractors and an intense light such as laparoscopic fiber-optic light may be required.
- Once the peritoneum is visualized, it is grasped by two artery forceps and incised in-between by scissors, allowing entrance to the peritoneal cavity.
- A blunt tip balloon trocar or an ordinary trocar can be used, provided the wound is completely sealed to prevent air leak.
- The CO_2 is insufflated at high flow, the other port sites are marked and the trocars are inserted with intra-abdominal pressure of at least 15 mmHg.
- The retroperitoneum is always accessed by an open technique.

BALLOON DILATOR

- The retroperitoneal space is primarily formed by finger dissection, allowing insertion of the balloon dilator to achieve optimal dilatation (Figure 3.3).

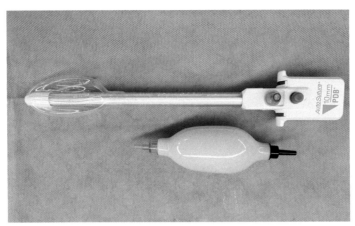

Figure 3.3 Balloon dilator (non-inflated) with the pump device.

- Around 400 mL of air (35–40 pumps) is sufficient for creating an adequate space.
- An obvious tense bulge will be seen externally at the same area because of the balloon.
- Inflation of the balloon can also be performed under laparoscopic vision through the transparent obturator (optiview trocar).
- This will allow space inspection to ensure correct placement and rule out peritoneal injury.

TROCARS

- In da Vinci Xi robot, 8-mm reusable metallic trocars are used and inserted, guided by the black line markings on the cannula shaft (Figure 3.4).

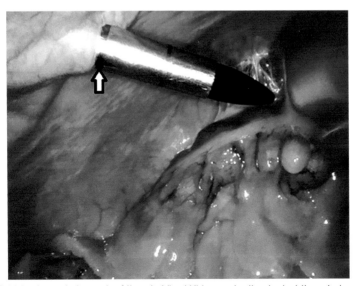

Figure 3.4 The fat black mark (arrow) of the da Vinci Xi trocar is situated at the abdominal wall.

- Laparoscopic trocars are disposable with bladeless fascial dilating tips, and various sizes are available (Figure 3.5).

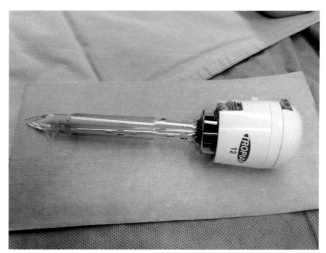

Figure 3.5 A 12-mm laparoscopic trocar with bladeless dilating tip.

TROCAR INSERTIONS

- Skin incision is made slightly larger than the trocar diameter to avoid forcible insertion resulting in overshooting causing intraperitoneal injuries.
- The intra-abdominal (pneumoperitoneum) pressure should be adequate and preferably kept at 15 mmHg during insertion.
- The trocar is firmly held and supported by the palm of the hand and controlled by the index finger on the shaft to prevent overshooting (Figure 3.6).

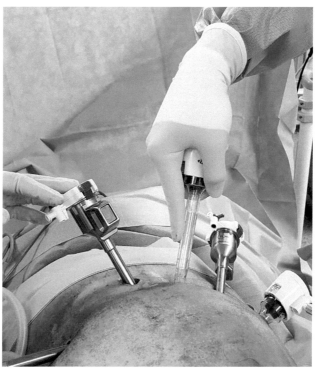

Figure 3.6 Trocar handling during insertion.

- The abdominal wall is stabilized by towel clips and the trocar is inserted perpendicular to the wall by screwing movement, applying a steady downward force.

- Once the trocar gives away and the resistance disappears, the obturator is removed and the cannula valve is opened to hear the hiss of air, confirming the correct placement.
- The gas insufflator tube is connected with high flow.
- The laparoscope is introduced through the first port to rule out any injuries secondary to the access, rule out intestinal adhesions and assess the entry sites of the next ports.
- The exact trocar site on the skin can be confirmed by visualizing the finger or trocar tip impressions internally through the scope.
- The intestine can be retracted away from the entry point using a fan retractor.

If omental or bowel adhesions are present at a trocar entry site, then adhesiolysis is performed before insertion.

- The additional trocars are placed under laparoscopic visualization, minimizing inadvertent vascular or visceral injuries.
- Once the tip of the obturator penetrates the peritoneum, the trocar is slid toward the target organ (Figure 3.7).

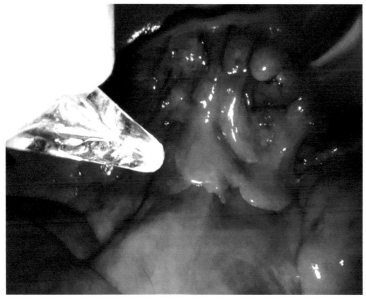

Figure 3.7 Sliding the trocar toward the target organ once the obturator tip penetrates the peritoneum.

- The obturator is removed once the distal part of the sheath is visualized, and the cannula is further adjusted.

A right-angled clamp can be applied against the abdominal wall around the trocar tip to facilitate a safe insertion, as during the introduction of the 5 mm liver traction trocar.

BALLOON TROCAR

- The open access wound is usually quiet large for the trocar's diameter, allowing air to leak.
- To secure the trocar in place and minimize the leakage, a 10-mm blunt tip balloon cannula with smaller reducers is used (Figure 3.8).
- The tract is sealed between the balloon and a sponge, which is tightened by a plastic locker on top of it.
- Because the balloon trocar is fixed in place at the abdominal wall, the access site should be carefully decided according to the distance from the target area.

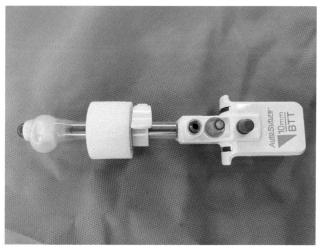

Figure 3.8 Balloon trocar. Note the sponge collar with a locker on top of it.

PORT CONFIGURATION

- The ports are placed around 15–20 cm from the target organ.
- The triangulation principle in port placement is applied in laparoscopic procedures, so the working ports form a triangle with the camera (scope) (Figure 3.9).

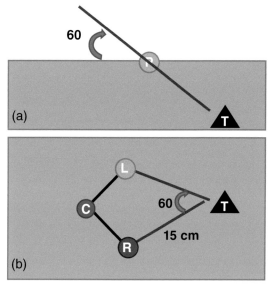

Figure 3.9 The triangulation principle and baseball diamond concept in port placement in relation to the target organ (T). Note the 60° elevation angle in (a) and manipulation angle in (b).

- In relation to the target organ, the trocar configurations will display the diamond baseball concept in the position of the ports.
- These principles are essential for achieving the best task performance efficiency by providing accurate working angles.
- The optimal manipulation angle between the instruments at the target tissue level is around 60°.
- This will correspond to the elevation angle of about 60° between the instrument and the abdomen axis of the patient.
- The trocars are placed around 7 cm apart.

The farther the trocars are, it is less likely for the instruments to clash, but the wider the shoulder angles, it causes more fatigue to surgeon.

- The sectorization principle where the camera is positioned lateral to the working ports may also be applied in certain steps of the procedure, e.g., prostatectomy (Figure 3.10).

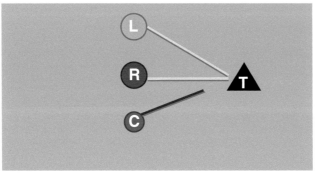

Figure 3.10 The sectorization principle in port placement. The camera port (C) is lateral to the working left- and right-hand ports (L, R). *Abbreviation:* T, target organ.

PORT SITE CLOSURE

- In the transperitoneal approach, port sites that are more than 10 mm, are closed by using the Carter Thomason suture pass device using a 1/0 vicryl stitch (Figure 3.11).

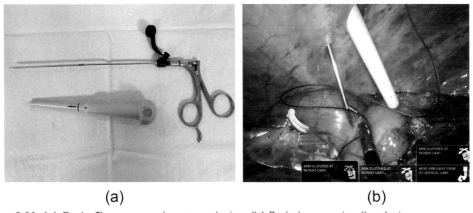

(a)   (b)

Figure 3.11 (a) Carter Thomason suture pass device. (b) Port closure using the device.

- The closure includes the fascial layers of the abdominal wall in addition to the peritoneum.
- The large wounds of specimen retrieval and the access site of the retroperitoneal approach are closed by continuous hand suturing using a 1/0 vicryl stitch.

Laparoscopic Urologic Surgery

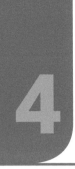

4 Transperitoneal Laparoscopic Radical Prostatectomy

POSITION

- The patient is positioned supine for draping and trocar, insertion.
- The rest of the procedure is performed in the Trendelenburg position with the legs straight and both arms alongside the body (Figure 4.1).
- Straps and adhesives are applied to support and stabilize the patient.
- A flatus tube is introduced into the rectum and a urethral catheter is inserted in the sterile draped field.

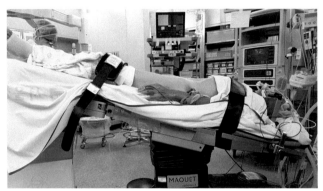

Figure 4.1 Trendelenburg position. The patient is strapped and supported; pressure areas are padded; electrocautery is connected; flatus tube is inserted; and intermittent pneumatic calf compression device and elastic stocking are applied. Arms should be wrapped and padded to the patient's side.

PORT INSERTION

- In the supine position, the Veress needle is introduced through a 15-mm hemi-circumferential incision around the right border of the umbilicus.

Confirmation of correct Veress needle passage and position is explained in Chapter 3, Section 1 "Basic Instrumentation".

- Pneumoperitoneum is created to 15 mmHg for trocar insertion, after which it is set down to 12 mmHg throughout the procedure.

Access can also be obtained by using the open (Hasson) technique or by direct vision using an optiview trocar with the laparoscope.

DOI: 10.1201/b22928-6

- An 11-mm trocar is inserted at the Veress needle site and a 10-mm, 30° lens laparoscope is introduced to assess the following:

  - Veress needle and port entry area for injuries
  - Presence of adhesions
  - Main landmarks and critical structures
  - Entry sites for next ports

- Another four 11-mm trocars are inserted, about 15 cm from the symphysis pubis in a fan (hemi-circular) shape toward the pelvis with around 7 cm in-between (Figure 4.2).

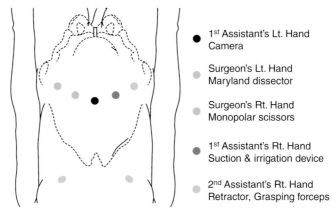

Figure 4.2 Diagram of the port configurations, the surgeon's position and instruments being used.

For the far lateral ports, the intestine may need to be retracted medially during trocar insertion to avoid bowel injury.

OPERATING ROOM SETUP AND SURGEON POSITIONS

- The surgeon stands at the left side of the patient and the first assistant stands at the right side of the patient, holding the camera and using the right-side ports for assistance.
- A second assistant stands at the right side of the patient, using the far lateral port and taking care of catheter manipulation, catheter change and bladder filling.
- The operating room is set up to facilitate a smooth flow of surgery (Figure 4.3).

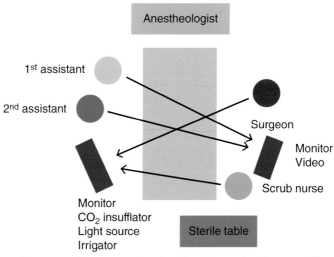

Figure 4.3 Diagram of the operation room setup showing the surgical team position in relation to the patient, monitors and the accessory machines.

STEP-BY-STEP SURGERY

ADHESIOLYSIS

- The intestine is retracted cranially from the pelvis and bowel adhesions at the pelvic side wall or at the dissection area are lysed if present (Figure 4.4).

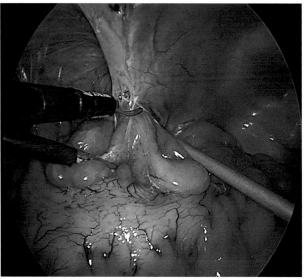

Figure 4.4 Releasing the sigmoid colon adhesions at the left pelvic side wall.

> In addition to the Trendelenburg position, releasing the adhesions will empty the pelvis and provide a safe dissection area.

DROPPING THE BLADDER AND ENTERING THE RETZIUS SPACE

- The surgeon uses a Maryland forceps through a left-side port and scissors through the right para-median port.
- The right medial umbilical ligament is retracted down just distal to the umbilicus by the left Maryland.
- The peritoneum is incised horizontally using monopolar scissors just lateral and parallel to the ligament (Figure 4.5).

> The dissection is carried out through the areolar tissue plane on the peritoneum and care is taken not to superficially dissect the transversalis fascia anteriorly (Figure 4.6).

- The assistant further retracts down the peritoneal flap with a suction device while clearing up the smoke.
- The same step is performed for the left medial umbilical ligament using the two left-sided ports (Sectorization).

> The urachus is not transected and kept attached to the anterior abdominal wall. This may prevent a fall of intestine into the surgical field.

- The peritoneum is incised as an inverted V shape following the medial umbilical ligaments until crossing the vas deference medial to the internal inguinal ring (Figure 4.7).

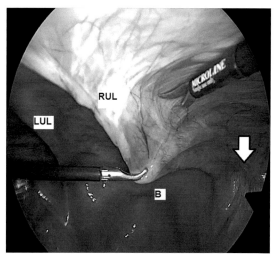

Figure 4.5 Anterior peritoneal dissection. Internal inguinal ring (arrow). *Abbreviations*: B, bladder; LUL, left medial umbilical ligament; RUL, right medial umbilical ligament.

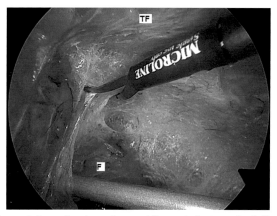

Figure 4.6 Anterior peritoneal dissection is performed through the areolar fatty plane avoiding the transversalis fascia (TF) anteriorly. *Abbreviation*: F, extraperitoneal fat.

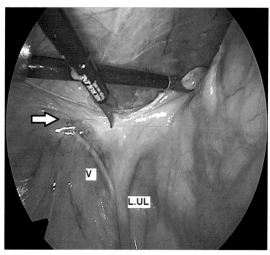

Figure 4.7 Peritoneal incision from urachus until the vas (V) laterally, medial to internal inguinal ring (arrow). *Abbreviation*: L.UL, left medial umbilical ligament.

> Dissecting far lateral to the medial umbilical ligament and internal inguinal ring landmarks may injure the inferior epigastric vessels.

- The vas is isolated, clipped by M size Hem-o-lok and transected by monopolar scissors (Figure 4.8).

> Ligating the vas at this level will obviate the need to clip it posterior to bladder neck at a later step. This will avoid the presence of a foreign body near the urethrovesical anastomosis.

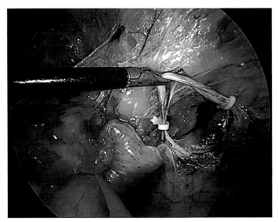

Figure 4.8 Isolation, clip ligation and division of the right vas deference.

- The dissection in the plane of gray, loose areolar tissue is continued until the bony pelvis, anterior to the bladder and prostate (Retzius space) (Figure 4.9).

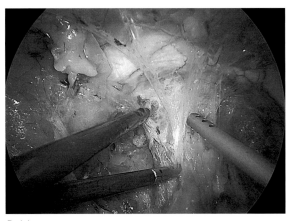

Figure 4.9 Entering the Retzius space.

- From the level of clipped vas, the lateral bladder wall is dissected off the lateral pelvic wall fat through a relatively avascular plane by blunt and sharp dissection (Figure 4.10).

Take care to avoid injury to the ureter, external iliac vessels and obturator nerve on the lateral pelvic wall.

> Releasing the lateral bladder walls from the pelvic side wall will provide extra bladder mobility and facilitate a tension-free vesicourethral anastomosis.

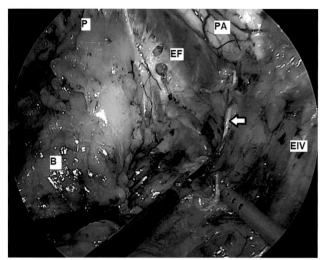

Figure 4.10 Lateral bladder wall dissection. Obturator nerve (arrow). *Abbreviations*: B, bladder; EF, endopelvic fascia; EIV, external iliac vein; PA, pubic arch; P, prostate (right side).

DEFATTING THE PROSTATE AND ENDOPELVIC FASCIA

- The fat overlaying the endopelvic fascia and prostate is swept off and rolled medially and proximally toward the bladder.

Take care to avoid injury to the accessory pudendal artery which, if present, may be identified laterally on the endopelvic fascia (Figure 4.11).

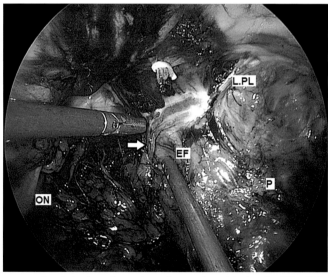

Figure 4.11 Accessory pudendal artery (arrow) on the endopelvic fascia (EF). *Abbreviations*: LPL, left puboprostatic ligament; ON, left obturator nerve; P, prostate.

- The superficial dorsal vein is identified in the fat between the two puboprostatic ligaments. It is isolated, cauterized and transected (Figure 4.12).
- The fat is excised and kept at the left iliac fossa to be included later with the specimen.

The prostatic fat is light and easily removed compared to adherent fat of the bladder, demarcating the vesicoprostatic junction.

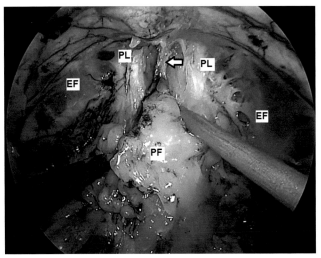

Figure 4.12 Defatting of the prostate and endopelvic fascia. Superficial dorsal vein (arrow). *Abbreviations*: EF, endopelvic fascia; PF, prostatic fat; PL, puboprostatic ligaments.

Venous bleeding encountered while removing the prostatic fat at the level of the bladder neck is usually from the superficial dorsal vein extension.

The purpose of removing prostatic and endopelvic fat:

1. Demarcating the vesicoprostatic junction
2. Accurate opening of endopelvic fascia lateral to prostate
3. Visualizing the puboprostatic ligament overlying the dorsal vascular complex (DVC)
4. Defining the prostatic contour
5. Facilitating the dissection of bladder neck
6. For histopathology examination

OPENING THE ENDOPELVIC FASCIA

- The endopelvic fascia is incised lateral to the prostate and just distal to the bladder neck (Figure 4.13).
- The levator muscle within the layers of endopelvic fascia is peeled off the prostate and swept toward the pelvic wall without cautery (Figure 4.14).

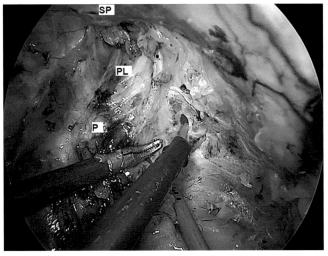

Figure 4.13 Opening of the left endopelvic fascia. *Abbreviations*: P, prostate; PL, puboprostatic ligament; SP, symphysis pubis. Note the medial retraction of the prostate.

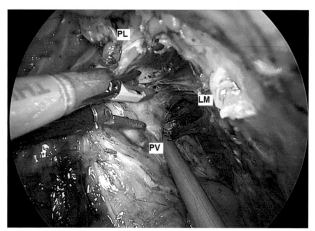

Figure 4.14 Peeling off the levator muscle from the prostate. *Abbreviations*: LM, levator muscle; PL, puboprostatic ligament; PV, periprostatic veins.

Take care to avoid the large dilated veins on the lateral wall of the prostate and medial to the endopelvic fascial incision.

- Endopelvic fascia incision is extended toward the prostatic apex where the puboprostatic ligament is transected and apical muscular attachment is identified and released (Figure 4.15).

> Puboprostatic ligament division will allow visualizing the prostatic apex, DVC, apical muscular attachment.

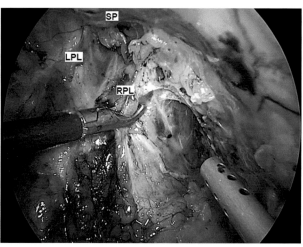

Figure 4.15 Transection of right puboprostatic ligament (RPL). *Abbreviations*: LPL, left puboprostatic ligament; SP, symphysis pubis.

- The distal apical lateral muscle attachment may contain a small vessel. It is coagulated and transected on the prostatic surface by an energy device and swept off to the pelvic wall (Figure 4.16).

> Releasing the apical muscular attachment will clearly visualize the lateral wall of the DVC and facilitate accurate ligation.

The same steps are followed for the other side.

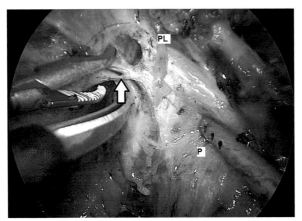

Figure 4.16 Release of apical muscular attachment containing a blood vessel (arrow). *Abbreviations*: LP, left puboprostatic ligament; P, prostate.

DVC LIGATION

- Once the puboprostatic ligament is incised and the apex is cleared from the muscular attachment, the DVC will be visualized.
- A 31-mm MH-1, 1/2 circle needle on a 20-cm PDS stitch is used for DVC ligation.
- The needle is horizontally oriented with its curve parallel to the pubic arch (Figure 4.17).

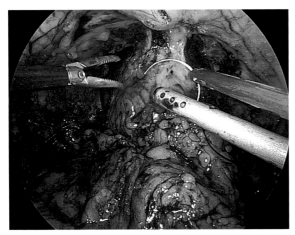

Figure 4.17 The orientation of the needle for deep vascular complex (DVC) ligation.

- The needle is introduced at a right angle through the plane between DVC and the urethra from right to left using wrist rotation (pronation movement).
- For optimum exposure during needle introduction, the surgeon's left hand retracts the prostatic apex to the left while the assistant retracts on the bladder neck level (Figure 4.18).
- Once the needle pierces the right side, the left side is exposed by the assistant suction device retracting on the prostatic apex to the right and the needle exit is adjusted (Figure 4.19).
- The needle is removed with its curve to avoid DVC injury and bleeding.
- The DVC is ligated as a figure of 8 with a slip-knot to ensure a tight closure (Figure 4.20).
- A bunching stitch is performed to include a wide bladder detrusor apron on the prostate base just distal to the vesicoprostatic junction.

The bladder bunching stitch at the base of the prostate will facilitate the incision through the detrusor muscle during bladder neck transection. It may also decrease bothersome back bleeders from the DVC.

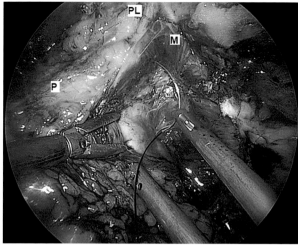

Figure 4.18 Needle is introduced perpendicular to the right side of the DVC. Note the retraction. *Abbreviations*: M, apical muscles; P, prostate; PL, transected puboprostatic ligament.

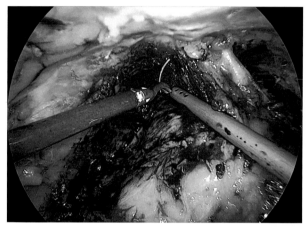

Figure 4.19 Needle exit from the left side of DVC. Note the suction probe retraction.

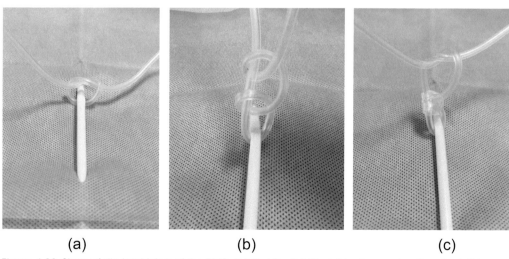

(a) (b) (c)

Figure 4.20 Steps of slip-knot tying of the DVC. (a) First tie. (b) Straightening and pulling the left long thread to slip down and tighten the knot after second tie. (c) Third tie to secure the knot.

Ways for defining the bladder neck:

1. Margin between loose fat of the prostate and the adherent fat of the bladder.
2. The consistency difference of firm prostate and soft bladder.
3. Bladder neck outlined by the catheter balloon under traction.
4. The crossing fibers of the two puboprostatic ligaments meet at the vesicoprostatic junction (variable between patients).

- The bladder neck is transected just proximal to the bunching stitch using an energy device (ultrasonic shears) or monopolar scissors (Figure 4.21).

Using ultrasonic shears for bladder neck division ensures the transection at the vesicoprostatic junction, because it will resettle on the correct plane even when it grasps the prostate.

- Gentle down traction on the bladder with a left-hand Maryland, and assistant suction device will facilitate the bladder neck transection by the energy device and will visualize the muscle fibers.

Preserving the bladder neck is not mandatory, and proximal transection is less hazardous than having a positive margin. Furthermore, wider bladder neck will facilitate the laparoscopic vesicourethral anastomosis in the pelvis.

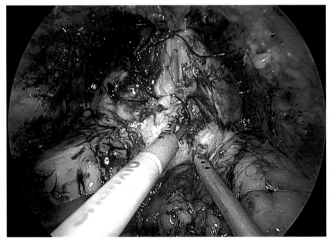

Figure 4.21 Transection of the bladder neck muscle fibers using ultrasonic shears with bladder down traction. The prostate and endopelvic fascia are completely defatted.

In a large prostate or large median lobe, the configuration of the bladder neck may differ and incision site is changed accordingly.

Reviewing preoperative MRI images is important to estimate the prostatic size and rule out asymmetric configuration.

- Once the anterior bladder neck is transected, the urethral catheter is retracted anteriorly by a thread introduced by a Suture passer needle just above the symphysis pubis (Figure 4.22).

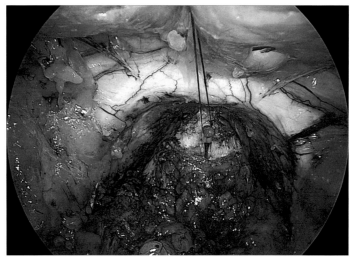

Figure 4.22 Foley catheter traction to anterior abdominal wall.

- The external part of the urethral catheter is fixed to the patient drape.

The use of a traction thread will omit the need for an additional trocar.

> The outward and upward traction of the prostate by the urethral catheter will define the prostatic contour and facilitate the dissection.

- The posterior bladder neck mucosa is horizontally incised by monopolar scissors and the dissection is continued deep posteriorly on the contour of prostatic gland (Figure 4.23).

> The lateral walls of bladder neck with perivesical fat are thinned out and flattened to easily facilitate the posterior mucosal incision and for further deep dissection.

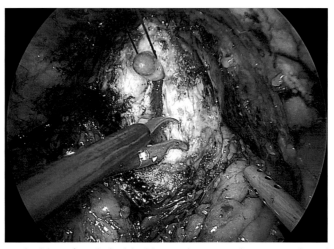

Figure 4.23 Transverse incision of posterior bladder neck mucosa by monopolar scissors.

- Gentle pressure on the anterior bladder neck will expose the posterior bladder neck wall and visualize the prostatic borders.
- If a median lobe is encountered, the overlying mucosa is incised and the plane between the lobe and bladder wall is identified and dissected following the prostatic contour.
  - This is facilitated by anterior traction of the median lobe by locking grasper of the second assistant with a posterior countertraction to the bladder neck by the first assistant.

> Assessing the bladder wall thickness during posterior dissection is critical to avoid buttonholing of the bladder or injuring the ureteric orifices.

- The dissection is continued until the thin posterior longitudinal muscle fibers of the bladder neck are transected (Figure 4.24).

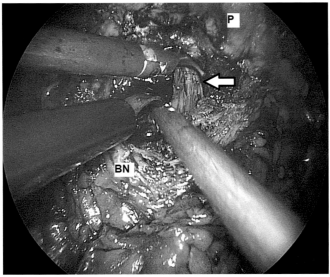

Figure 4.24 Longitudinal muscle fibers (arrow) transection. *Abbreviations*: BN, bladder neck; P, prostate with anterior traction by catheter.

VAS DEFERENCE, SEMINAL VESICLE AND PROSTATIC PEDICLE

- The vasa and seminal vesicles are identified posterior to the longitudinal muscle fiber layers.

> Reviewing the preoperative sagittal images will provide key information about the depth of the vasa and seminal vesicles (Figure 4.25).

- The vas (one side) is grasped and the blood vessels and connective tissue attachment are cauterized and peeled off.
- The assistant's posterior countertraction by the suction device opens the space and aids the dissection (Figure 4.26).
- The vas is transected and the distal stump is retracted further anteriorly by the second assistant locking grasper to improve the seminal vesicle exposure.
- The Foley catheter traction is released.
- The seminal vesicle just lateral to the vas is grasped and dissected by sweeping off and cauterizing the blood vessels and connective tissue attachment (Figure 4.27).

To avoid any collateral thermal injuries to the posterolateral neurovascular bundle (NVB), electrocautery, if needed, is minimized and applied directly on the surface wall of the vas deference and seminal vesicles.

41

> Applying clips to small vessels of the seminal vesicles and vas deference is not required. This will avoid the presence of foreign bodies near the urethrovesical anastomosis.

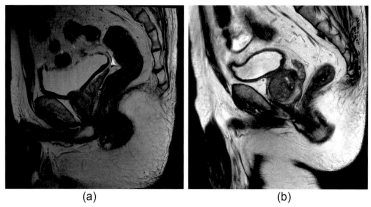

(a)   (b)

Figure 4.25 Sagittal sections of T2 MRI, showing the relationship between the bladder neck and seminal vesicle estimating the depth of dissection. (a) Shallow. (b) Deep.

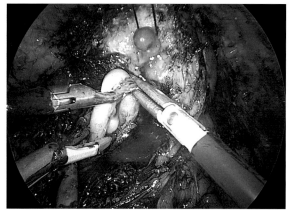

Figure 4.26 Dissection of the left vas deference. The seminal vesicle is just seen. Note the down traction by suction probe and the upward traction of the vas by locking grasper.

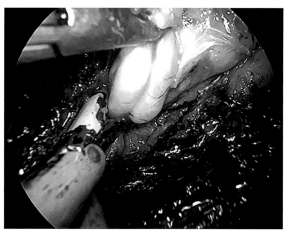

Figure 4.27 Dissection of the left seminal vesicle.

- The seminal vesicle is dissected until its junction with the prostate and with further anterior traction; the Denonvilliers' fascia will be clearly seen stretched posteriorly (Figure 4.28).
- The prostatic pedicle at the posterolateral edge of the prostate is dissected, thinned and clipped using an L-size Hem-o-lok just near the prostate.

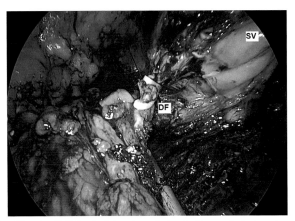

Figure 4.28 Denonvilliers' fascia (DF) is stretched posterior to the anteriorly retracted left seminal vesicle (SV). The left prostatic pedicle is clipped.

- Once the pedicle is clipped, it is divided by cold scissors close to the prostate.
- Denonvilliers' fascia attachment to the prostate is opened horizontally just posterior to the junction between seminal vesicle and prostate aiming for the intra-facial plane (if nerve sparing was planned).

No electrocautery is used in this area.

- The intra-fascial plane dissection between the Denonvilliers' fascia and prostate is continued distally toward the apex (Figure 4.29).

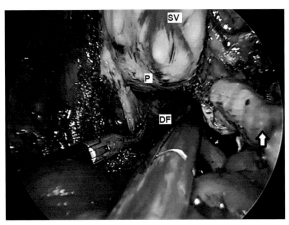

Figure 4.29 Intra-fascial dissection between the Denonvilliers' fascia (DF) and prostatic capsule (P). Right seminal vesicle (arrow). *Abbreviation*: SV, Left seminal vesicle.

- The assistant provides a posterior downward countertraction on the Denonvilliers' fascia.

Take care to avoid deep posterior dissection or excessive downward pressure, which may perforate the fascia into the rectum.

- The Denonvilliers' and prostatic fascia are released from the prostatic capsule by meticulous blunt and sharp dissection.
- To prevent capsular injury because of excessive traction, the small perforating vessels or fibrous attachment to the prostate are cauterized and/or divided.

NERVE SPARING

The NVB lies between the prostatic fascia and levator fascia layers.

- For nerve sparing, the dissection should be performed in the intra-facial plane between the prostatic capsule and prostatic fascia.
- The posterior intra-fascial plane already created above the Denonvilliers' fascia is connected by a right-angled dissector to the lateral plane.
- From the posterolateral edge (horn) of the prostate, at the level of divided prostatic pedicle, the levator and prostatic fascia are peeled off from the prostatic capsule using cold scissors.
- Blunt and sharp dissection is continued in anterolateral direction until the puboprostatic ligament on the prostatic apex (Figure 4.30).

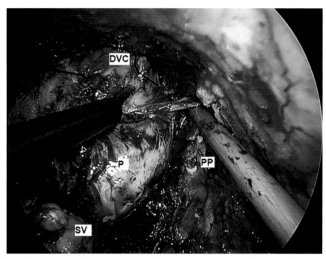

Figure 4.30 NVB dissection by peeling the prostatic and levator fascia from the prostate (P) using cold scissors. *Abbreviations*: DVC, ligated deep vascular complex; PP, clipped prostatic pedicle; SV, right seminal vesicle.

- The dissection is facilitated by contralateral countertraction of the prostate by the second assistant locking grasper on the seminal vesicle.
- Bleeding from the dilated periprostatic veins may occur. It usually stops spontaneously, avoiding unnecessary electrocautery.

The same steps are followed for the other side.

DVC AND URETHRAL DIVISION

- The DVC is divided at the level of the prostatic apex using hot monopolar scissors until the level of the urethra.
- The assistant should provide irrigation and suction of blood, fluid and gas to clear the field of vision.
- The urethra is divided by cold scissors and the urethral catheter is partially withdrawn by the assistant to complete the urethral transection (Figure 4.31).
- Posteriorly a small apical prostatic lip may be encountered extending distally.

Avoiding positive margin at the apex should not significantly compromise the urethral length.

- Rectaurethralis and remaining Denonvilliers' fascia attachments are gently and carefully released (Figure 4.32).

Rectal tenting during removal of the prostate due to posterior apical attachments avoids risking injury to the rectum.

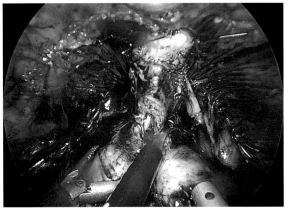

Figure 4.31 Sharp division of the urethra by cold scissors.

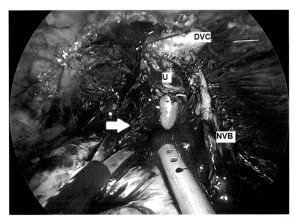

Figure 4.32 Releasing the residual rectourethralis (arrow) attachment. *Abbreviations*: DVC, deep vascular complex; NVB, neurovascular bundle; U, urethra.

- The excised prostate and the previously resected prostatic fat are introduced into an endo-catch bag.
- The bag is closed and the thread is clipped near the bag to ensure the closure.

HEMOSTASIS

- The dissection area at the prostatic bed and Denonvilliers' fascia above the rectum is cleaned by suction irrigation (Figure 4.33).
- Active bleeding, if present, is secured by clips, suturing or by selective coagulation and a hemostatic agent such as FloSeal is applied on the dissection area.

Pelvic lymphadenectomy if indicated is performed at this step.

POSTERIOR RECONSTRUCTION (MODIFIED ROCCO STITCH)

- The FloSeal is washed out and hemostasis is reassessed.
- Active bleeders at the NVB region are clipped or sutured rather than cauterized.
- Posterior reconstruction incorporates the longitudinal muscles of the posterior bladder neck and Denonvilliers' fascia to the periurethral tissue of the rectourethralis muscle (Figure 4.34).
- Suturing is performed by a 15-cm, 3/0 V-Loc stitch on 1/2 circle using a 17-mm CV-23 needle from left to right, cephalo-caudal direction in three running stitches.

The posterior reconstruction facilitates a tension-free vesicourethral anastomosis and may enhance early recovery of post-prostatectomy incontinence.

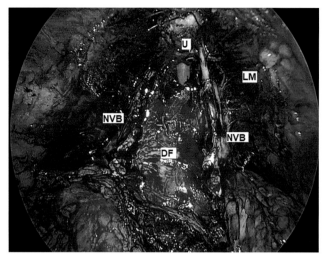

Figure 4.33 Prostatic bed *Abbreviations*: DF, Denonvilliers' fascia; LM, levator muscle; NVB, neurovascular bundles; U, urethra.

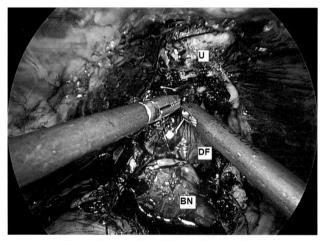

Figure 4.34 Posterior reconstruction. *Abbreviations*: BN, longitudinal fibers posterior to bladder neck; DF, Denonvilliers' fascia; U, urethra.

VESICO-URETHRAL ANASTOMOSIS

To achieve the optimal angle for easy and accurate suturing, the surgeon uses the left-most trocar for the left needle driver and the right pararectal trocar for the right needle driver.

> Visual field orientation is essential for correct and precise anastomosis. Camera rotation is avoided and the symphysis pubis should always be oriented at 12 o'clock position.

- The anastomosis begins at 5 o'clock position by using the same V-Loc stitch of the posterior reconstruction, which ends just to the right of the urethra.
- The anastomosis is performed by continuous running suturing starting first on the left side then on the right.

> For every urethral stitch, the second assistant should manipulate the catheter tip in/out to open the urethra and guide the surgeon's needle (Figure 4.35).

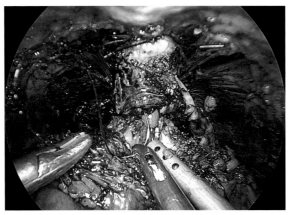

Figure 4.35 The needle is guided by the Foley catheter.

- After making the bladder neck 6 o' clock stitch, the suture line is tightened, approximating the bladder to the urethra.

Throughout the anastomosis, the suturing is always outside-in at the bladder and inside-out at the urethra.

For precise left-side suturing from 7 to 11 o'clock:

* The bladder outside-in is performed by the left hand.
* The urethral inside-out is performed by the right hand (Figure 4.36).

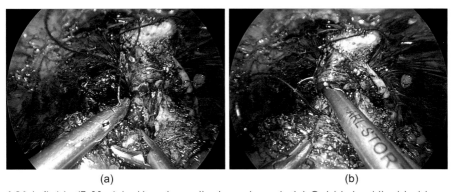

(a)   (b)

Figure 4.36 Left side (7–11 o'clock) vesicourethral anastomosis. (a) Outside-in at the bladder neck by left hand. (b) Inside-out at the urethra by right hand.

Everting bladder mucosa is not a must; however, including a few millimeters from the mucosal edge is crucial and sufficient to ensure a mucosa to mucosa anastomosis.

- With the suction device, the assistant exposes the bladder neck wall and clears the field and urethra from blood.
- Once left-side anastomosis reaches 11 o'clock, a similar V-Loc 3/0 stitch is introduced to start suturing the right side from 4 o'clock to 12 o'clock.

For right-side precise suturing from 4 o'clock to 12 o'clock:

* The bladder outside-in is performed by the right hand.
* The urethral inside-out is performed by the left hand (Figure 4.37).

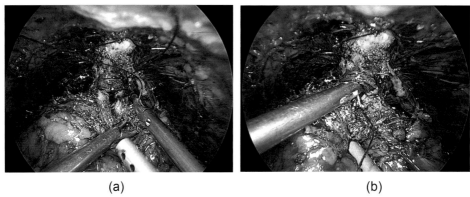

(a)   (b)

Figure 4.37 Right-side (4–12 o'clock) vesicourethral anastomosis. (a) Outside-in at the bladder neck by right hand. (b) Inside-out at the urethra by left hand.

> To avoid tearing of the urethral wall while tightening the anastomosis line, the stitch is pulled straight, perpendicular to the wall, which can be further supported by the instrument in the other hand.

- The residual anterior bladder neck gap is closed by the remaining right-side anastomosis stitch before tying it with the left one.
- Another V-Loc stitch may be required if the bladder neck gap is quiet large.

During this step, the second assistant should ensure that the urethral catheter is moving freely in and out without being entrapped by the stitch.

- The catheter is replaced by a new one because it may have been injured during needle guiding.
- The anastomosis integrity is assessed by filling the bladder to 150 ml of normal saline looking for fluid leakage. Unrecognized bladder wall injury or residual gaps can also be identified.

ANTERIOR RECONSTRUCTION

- Both sides of the bladder neck can be continuously sutured to the levator fascia and puboprostatic ligaments.
- A sling stitch for the bladder neck to the symphysis pubis is performed (Figure 4.38).

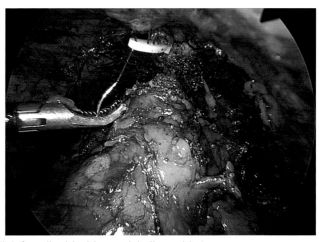

Figure 4.38 Sling stitch from the bladder neck to the pubic bone.

HEMOSTASIS, WOUND CLOSURE, DRAIN AND SPECIMEN EXTRACTION

- A hemostatic agent like Surgicel can be placed at the sides of the bladder neck, if necessary.
- Drain is inserted through a lateral port wound.
- Port sites are closed by 1/0 vicryl stitch using a Carter Thomason device.
- The specimen is removed through an extended camera port wound, which is closed in layers by hand suturing using 1/0 vicryl.

The detailed explanation along with figures for drain and closure is provided in Section 1.

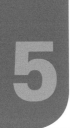

Transperitoneal Laparoscopic Radical Nephrectomy

POSITION

- The patient is positioned in a semi-lateral (60°) decubitus position with the abdomen at the table edge (Figure 5.1).
- Straps, adhesives and supporting pads are applied to stabilize the patient, and the urinary catheter is inserted before draping.

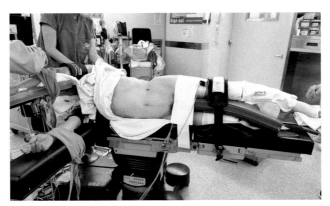

Figure 5.1 Semi-lateral decubitus position. The patient is strapped and supported; shoulder and pressure areas are padded; electrocautery is connected; urethral catheter is inserted; intermittent pneumatic calf compression device and elastic stocking are applied.

> The table is not flexed in a transperitoneal approach to avoid unnecessary rhabdomyolysis and postoperative neuromusculoskeletal pain.
>
> Table flexion may also decrease the working space by pushing the kidney close to the abdominal wall.

ACCESS

- In the lateral decubitus position, the Veress needle is introduced through a 1.5-cm, ipsilateral hemi-circumferential incision around the umbilicus (Figure 5.2).
- Gas flow can be increased once the correct position of the Veress needle is confirmed and 1 L is insufflated.

DOI: 10.1201/b22928-7

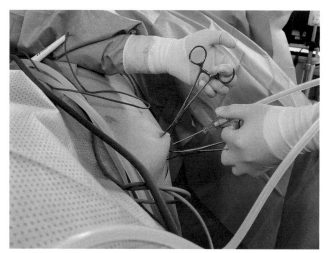

Figure 5.2 Veress needle insertion in lateral position. The abdomen is stabilized by two towel clips.

Confirmation of correct Veress needle passage and position is explained in Chapter 3, Section 1 "Basic Instrumentation".

- Pneumoperitoneum is created to 15 mmHg for trocar insertion, after which it is set down to 12 mmHg throughout the procedure.

Access can also be obtained by using the open (Hasson) technique or under direct vision using an optiview trocar with the laparoscope (Figure 5.3).

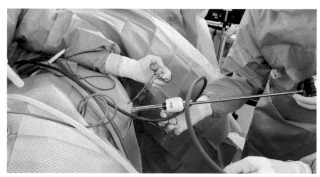

Figure 5.3 Optiview trocar insertion. Direct visualization of the abdominal layers using the scope through a visual obturator.

> For the left side, as more lateral bowel dissection is required to expose the renal hilum, a closed or open access (Hasson) is obtained at the ipsilateral pararectus muscle just caudal to the umbilicus.

PORT INSERTION

- An 11-mm trocar is inserted at the access site and a 10-mm, 30° lens laparoscope is introduced to assess:

  - Veress needle and port entry area for any injuries
  - Operation site and kidney outline
  - Presence of adhesions
  - Survey for abnormal anatomy or lesions
  - Entry sites of the next port

- If the open access wound obtained is quite large for the 11-mm trocar, then a blunt tip balloon trocar with a sponge collar is used to secure the port and minimize air leakage.
- Two 11-mm trocars are inserted applying the triangulation principle in port placement toward the kidney position (Figure 5.4).

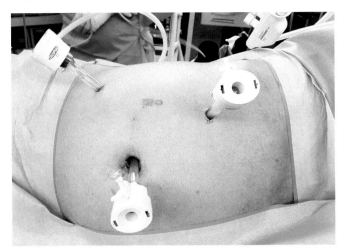

Figure 5.4 Trocar configurations applying the triangulation principle in port placement (for right kidney).

- A fourth trocar of 11 mm is inserted (*at a later step*) opposite of the camera, making a diamond-shaped configuration with other ports.

> Access site and port positions may vary depending on the patient's body habitus, tumor location, kidney anatomy, presence of adhesions and surgeon's preference. However, the principle of triangulation is applied, keeping the instruments at least 7 cm apart.

- For the right kidney, a 5-mm liver retraction trocar is inserted just inferior to the xiphoid process.

OPERATING ROOM SETUP AND SURGEON POSITIONS

- The operating room is set up to facilitate a smooth flow of surgery (Figure 5.5).
- The primary surgeon stands at the abdominal side of the patient.
- The first assistant stands caudal to the surgeon, toward the hip and a second assistant, if needed, stands at the back of the patient and opposite to the surgeon.

STEP-BY-STEP SURGERY

ADHESIOLYSIS AND LIVER RETRACTION

- Adhesiolysis is performed if bowel adhesions are present at the operation area or at the port entry sites.
- For the right kidney, the liver and gallbladder adhesions are released before introducing the retractor.
  - The right triangular ligament may need to be divided at this step (Figure 5.6).

> To avoid liver injury while inserting the retraction port, a right-angled grasper can be applied against the anterior abdominal wall around the entry point of the trocar (Figure 5.7).

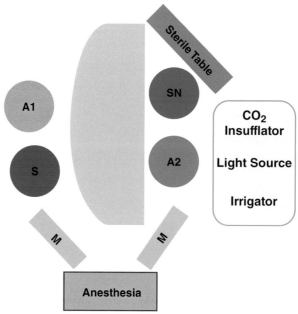

Figure 5.5 Diagram of the operation room setup showing the surgical team positions in relation to the patient, monitors (M) and the accessory machines. *Abbreviations*: A, assistants; S, primary surgeon; SN, scrub nurse.

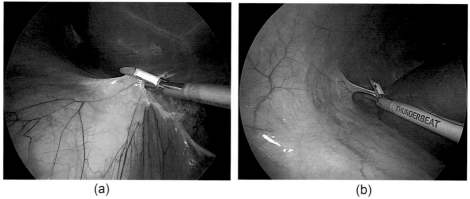

(a)   (b)

Figure 5.6 (a) Releasing the liver from adhesions. (b) Division of the right triangular ligament of the liver.

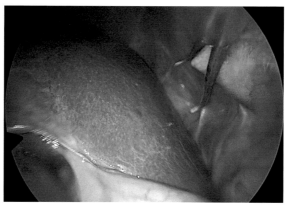

Figure 5.7 Using a right-angled grasper against the anterior abdominal wall during insertion of the 5-mm liver retraction trocar to avoid liver injury.

- Atraumatic non-crushing locking grasper is introduced and fixed to the diaphragm muscles supero-laterally (Figure 5.8).

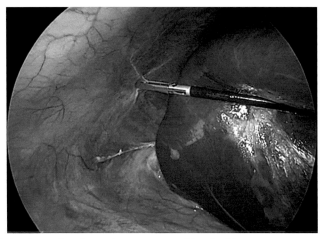

Figure 5.8 Self-retaining liver retraction using a non-crushing locking grasper.

COLON (DESCENDING OR ASCENDING) MOBILIZATION

- The peritoneum is opened at the white line of Toldt just lateral to the colon, reflecting the bowel medially (Figure 5.9).

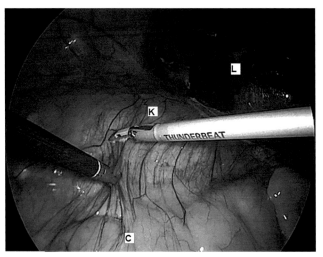

Figure 5.9 Opening of the peritoneum. *Abbreviations*: C, ascending colon; K, kidney; L, liver on traction.

- A plane between the white perinephric fat of Gerota and the yellow fat of the mesocolon is created by blunt and sharp dissection (Figure 5.10).

Meticulous and careful use of an energy device or monopolar scissors at this step is mandatory to avoid injuries to the colon or its mesentery.

- The dissection is carried out from the level of common iliac vessels inferiorly, up to the level of the colonic flexure and the diaphragm superiorly at the upper pole.

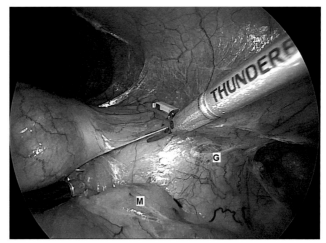

Figure 5.10 Dissection between the perinephric white fat of Gerota (G) and yellow fat of the mesocolon (M).

Oncologic surgery should be embryologic surgery. If the dissection is performed between the embryologically different planes, it should be easy and oncologically safe. Being an avascular plane, the bleeding should be minimal.

Dissecting the lateral Gerota attachment at this step must be avoided, as this will drop down the kidney medially and make the hilar dissection difficult.

The planes are opened carefully from superficial to deep, layer by layer, up and down along the line of dissection. Injuries or bleeding in deep and narrow spaces are difficult to manage due to inadequate exposure.

IN THE RIGHT SIDE

- The hepatorenal and posterior coronary ligaments of the liver are incised (Figure 5.11).

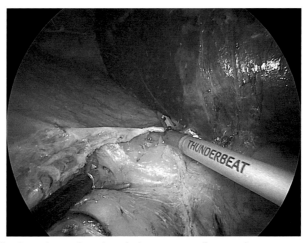

Figure 5.11 Incising the hepatorenal and posterior coronary ligaments.

The division of the hepatorenal and posterior coronary ligaments will expose the lateral wall of the vena cava above the adrenal gland, duodenum and renal hilum (Figure 5.12).

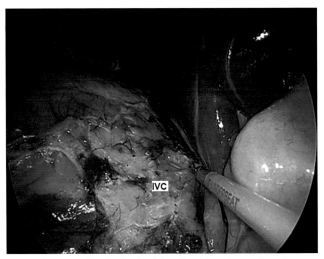

Figure 5.12 Infrahepatic IVC is visualized after incising the hepatorenal and coronary ligaments.

- After reflecting the colon medially, the duodenum is identified and Kocherized to reveal the anterior surface of the inferior vena cava (IVC) (Figure 5.13).

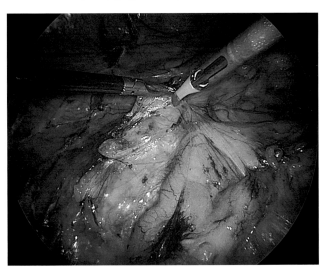

Figure 5.13 Kocherization of the duodenum.

Close contact to the duodenum by cautery or energy device blades must be avoided.

IN THE LEFT SIDE

- A slightly more extensive colon mobilization is required on the left side to include the splenic flexure, the spleen and the tail of pancreas.

Once the linorenal and splenocolic ligaments are divided, the spleen, pancreas and colon will drop and reflect medially. This decreases the risk of injury during later dissection of the hilum, adrenal gland and upper pole.

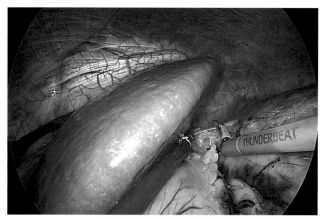

Figure 5.14 Incising the linorenal ligament.

- The incision of splenocolic, linorenal and phrenicocolic ligaments is carefully performed (Figure 5.14).

Take care to avoid spleen and stomach injury if extensive dissection of the left upper pole attachment is performed.

- The tail of pancreas is further released from the Gerota with the adrenal gland and upper pole of the kidney, taking care to avoid injury to the pancreatic tissue or the splenic vessels (Figure 5.15).

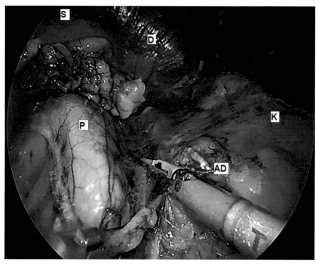

Figure 5.15 Releasing the tail of pancreas (P) from the left adrenal gland (AD) and upper pole kidney (K). The spleen (S) is dropped medially after incising the linorenal ligament. *Abbreviation*: D, diaphragm.

PSOAS MUSCLE, URETER AND GONADAL VESSELS

- Inferiorly, the anterior layer of Gerota's fascia is opened and dissected just lateral to IVC in the right side or to the aorta on the left (Figure 5.16).
- The gonadal vein and ureter are identified in the fibrofatty tissue above the psoas muscle.
- The vein is usually seen first anterior to the ureter.

In males, if only one tubular structure is identified then it is most likely the vein. To confirm, it can be followed toward the internal inguinal ring.

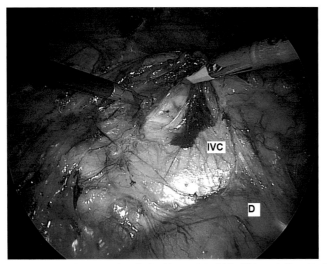

Figure 5.16 Opening the inferior Gerota's fascia just lateral to IVC. *Abbreviation*: D, duodenum.

- The gonadal vessels and the ureter are dissected and isolated and can be clipped and divided at this step or left until the pedicle is controlled.
- The assistant (fourth) port is inserted opposite to the camera, making a diamond-shaped configuration with the other ports, keeping at least 7 cm in-between (Figure 5.17).

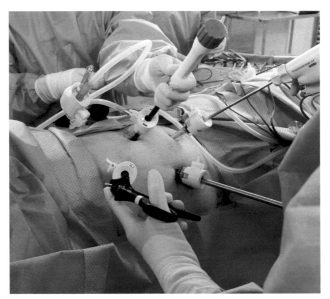

Figure 5.17 Diamond-shaped configuration with the fourth port (fan retractor).

- A fan retractor is introduced and the Gerota's fascia with the ureter-gonadal vein packet is retracted anterolaterally exposing the psoas muscle.

The anterolateral retraction of ureter-gonadal vein packet will stretch the medial and the posterior kidney attachments and will facilitate the dissection (Figure 5.18).

Take care to avoid excessive traction on the right gonadal vein to prevent avulsion injury at the level of the IVC.

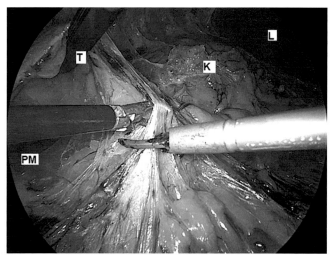

Figure 5.18 Release of anteromedial Gerota attachment. *Abbreviations*: K, right kidney; L, liver; PM, psoas muscle; T, anterolateral traction.

POSTEROMEDIAL DISSECTION

- Once the kidney is on traction, the posterior surface of Gerota will be clearly visualized.
- The posterior areolar attachment of Gerota to the psoas muscle is freed by blunt and sharp dissection.

Psoas fascia should be released intact to avoid muscle fiber exposure and unwanted bleeding.

- The medial Gerota attachment is dissected superficially layer by layer to avoid injuries to the gonadal vein or crossing vessels to the kidney and ureter.
- In the right side, the gonadal vein can be seen joining the IVC. It can be clipped and divided to avoid traction injury and significant bleeding (Figure 5.19).

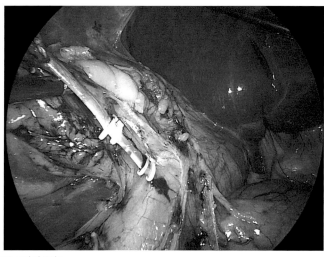

Figure 5.19 Right gonadal vein

- The fibro-lymphovascular tissue around the hilum is dissected with caution avoiding inadvertent vascular injuries.
- Bulky tissue attachment or small vessels can be clipped and transected by an energy device.
- Occasionally, hilar or para-aortic lymph nodes are encountered; they are either dissected and excised separately or resected en-bloc with the specimen.

THE PEDICLE

In the left side, the colon may fall back laterally on the field; it can be retracted to the abdominal wall by a stitch using a suture passer needle (Figure 5.20).

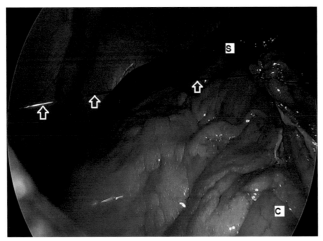

Figure 5.20 Descending colon (C) traction to anterior abdominal wall by PDS thread (arrows). *Abbreviation:* S, spleen.

- Once the Gerota attachment around the hilum is cleared, the renal vein can be clearly identified under tension because of traction.

The vena cava in the right and gonadal vein in the left can be used as guiding landmarks to the renal vein.

- The assistant's retractor position is adjusted to be just at the lower pole of the kidney, giving better exposure with gentle stretch of the pedicle.
- The anterior and inferior surfaces of the renal vein are cleared off the fibrofatty tissue (Figure 5.21).

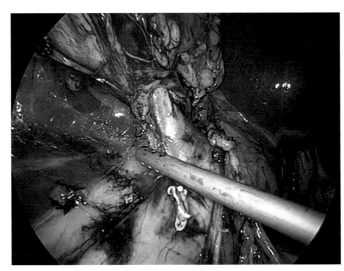

Figure 5.21 Right renal vein dissection.

- The left gonadal vein may need to be clipped and divided at this level if interfering with dissection.

- A lumbar vein joining the left renal vein may be identified, and is isolated, clipped by Hem-o-lok and divided (Figure 5.22).

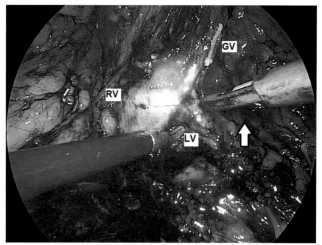

Figure 5.22 Dissecting and dividing the left lumbar vein (LV). Psoas muscle (arrow). *Abbreviations*: GV, clipped left gonadal vein; RV, left renal vein.

If the lumbar vein is not well controlled or injured during dissection, it may retract into the muscle and will be hard to catch and control.

Division of the left gonadal and lumbar vein will expose the renal artery.

- The lymphovascular tissue posterior to the renal vein is carefully dissected looking for the renal artery.
- The renal artery is identified by its pulsation or as a white wall tubular structure posterior the vein.
- The periarterial tissue is cleared to skeletonize the artery circumferentially using a Maryland or right-angled dissector and energy device.
- The tissue bands dissected off the artery are carefully coagulated and divided away from the vessel (Figure 5.23).

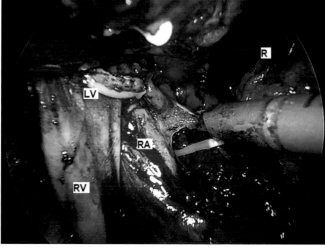

Figure 5.23 Dissection of the left renal artery (RA) using ultrasonic shears. *Abbreviations*: LV, clipped and divided lumbar vein; R, anterolateral retraction of the kidney; RV, left renal vein.

Laparoscopic Radical Nephrectomy

Suction probe can be utilized to facilitate identifying and dissecting the artery (Figure 5.24).

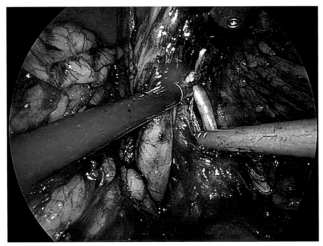

Figure 5.24 Dissection of the renal artery using a Maryland and right-hand suction probe.

If the renal artery is too deep for clipping, it can be retracted by a vessel loop or carefully grasped by the left-hand Maryland.

If the renal artery needs to be grasped and pulled out, the whole width of the artery should be included between the jaws of the grasper (Figure 5.25).

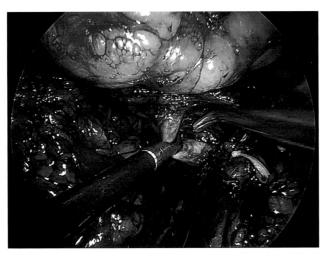

Figure 5.25 Right renal artery is completely grasped by a Maryland and a wide window is created using a right-angled dissector.

- The artery is clipped proximally by two L-size Hem-o-loks and two metallic titanium ligaclips and divided in-between the ligaclips using straight scissors (Figure 5.26).

If there is not enough space for multiple clips at the artery, the renal vein can be dissected and divided first after applying just one clip on the artery.

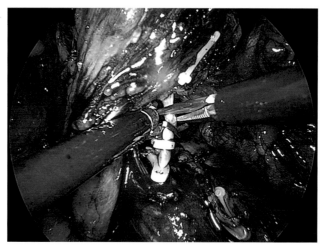

Figure 5.26 Clip ligation and division of left renal artery.

- Once the artery is divided, the vein should collapse, if not then look for another artery.

Reviewing the preoperative imaging study is critical to assess for early branching artery and to rule out multiple or accessory arteries (Figure 5.27).

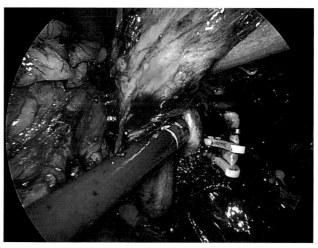

Figure 5.27 Dissecting a second renal artery. Revising the preoperative images is crucial to assess the vascular anatomy.

In a large and medially displaced left lower pole renal tumor, the superior mesenteric artery may be mistaken with the left renal artery.

- The renal vein is dissected and circumferentially freed from the fibrofatty tissue attachment creating an adequate window by a Maryland dissector and/or a right-angled dissector (Figure 5.28).
The left adrenal vein may be clipped and divided if interfering with dissection or vein ligation.

- A vessel loop is placed around the vein and retracted with a left-hand Maryland (Figure 5.29).
- The renal vein is clipped by two XL-size Hem-o-loks at the IVC side and one at the kidney side and divided in-between by straight scissors.

Correct method of clipping is explained in Section 1, Chapter 2.

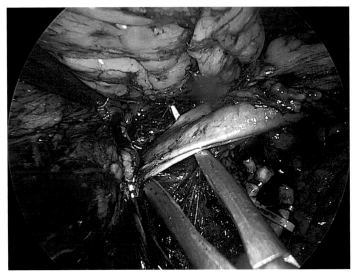

Figure 5.28 The renal vein is posteriorly dissected using a right-angled dissector and a wide window is created for safe ligation and division.

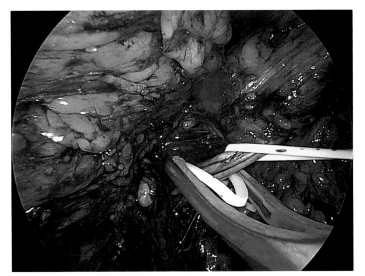

Figure 5.29 The right renal vein is retracted by a vessel loop and clipped using an XL Hem-o-lok. Note the angle of the clip applier is oriented to provide a space for next clips and safe margin for division.

Using a vessel loop to retract the renal vein will further shrink its wall and facilitate easy control and safe clipping.

ADRENAL GLAND PRESERVATION AND UPPER POLE DISSECTION

- The kidney is dropped down off the retractor and the Gerota's fascia is opened just above the divided renal vein.
- The perinephric fat is dissected upward on the anteromedial surface of the kidney (Figure 5.30).

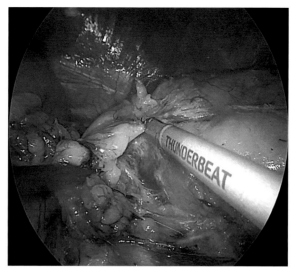

Figure 5.30 Separating the left adrenal gland from the upper pole of the kidney.

Take care to avoid injuries to aberrant vessels or other structures such as the pancreas, IVC and aorta medially.

- After adrenal separation, blunt and sharp dissection with an energy device is continued to free the upper pole.

To facilitate the left upper pole dissection, wide exposure can be achieved by a gentle superior-anterior traction of the spleen by the left-hand Maryland grasper (Figure 5.31).

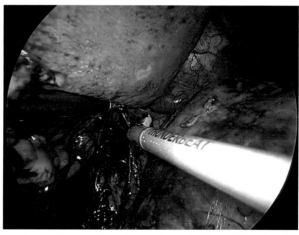

Figure 5.31 Superior-anterior traction of the spleen using a left-hand Maryland grasper during the dissection of the left upper pole residual attachment.

ADRENALECTOMY

- Occasionally, the adrenal gland removal with kidney is indicated, like in a huge upper pole tumor or when adrenal metastasis is suspected on imaging studies.
- On the right side, the extra Gerota dissection begins just lateral to the IVC.
- The adrenal vein is identified, clipped and divided just lateral to its origin at the IVC.
- On the left side, dissection begins medial to the adrenal vein and just lateral to the aorta.
- The left adrenal vein may not need to be ligated if the renal vein was proximally divided.

There may be no recognizable or sizable adrenal arteries, and dissecting them with an energy device is sufficient.

COMPLETION OF KIDNEY EXCISION

- Starting at the level of the divided ureter at inferior Gerota, the kidney is completely freed by blunt and sharp dissection from the lateral abdominal wall.
- The dissection is performed using an energy device through the avascular peritoneal plane between the Gerota's fascia and lateral peritoneal reflection (Figure 5.32).

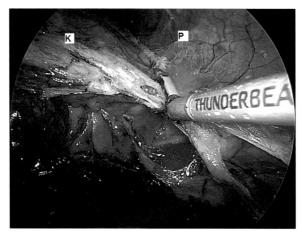

Figure 5.32 Completion of the left kidney (K) excision by dissecting off the Gerota from the lateral peritoneal reflection (P).

- The dissection is continued laterally until the upper pole is released off its remaining attachment.

DRAIN, SPECIMEN RETRIEVAL AND WOUND CLOSURE

- The kidney is introduced in an endo-catch bag (size depends on the specimen volume).
- The bag is closed and a clip is applied on the thread to ensure the closure.
- The dissection area is assessed for hemostasis and a drain is inserted if indicated.
- The port wounds are closed using a Carter Thomason suture pass device (Figure 5.33).
- The specimen is removed through a muscle-splitting Gibson or Pfannenstiel incision.

A detailed explanation of closure supported by figures are provided in Section 1, Chapter 3.

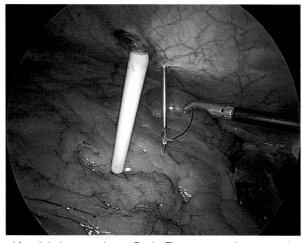

Figure 5.33 Port wound fascial closure using a Carter Thomason suture pass device.

Transperitoneal Laparoscopic Radical Nephroureterectomy

POSITION

- The patient is positioned in a semi-lateral (60°) decubitus position with the abdomen at the table edge (Figure 6.1).
- Straps, adhesives and supporting pads are applied to stabilize the patient, and a urethral catheter is inserted in the sterile draped field.

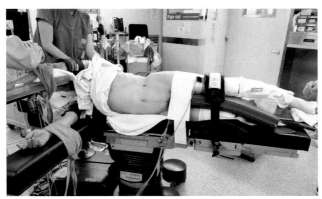

Figure 6.1 Semi-lateral decubitus position. The patient is strapped and supported; shoulder and pressure areas are padded; electrocautery is connected; urethral catheter is inserted; intermittent pneumatic calf compression device and elastic stocking are applied.

> The table is not flexed in a transperitoneal approach to avoid unnecessary rhabdomyolysis and postoperative neuromusculoskeletal pain.
>
> Table flexion may also decrease the working space by pushing the kidney close to the abdominal wall.

ACCESS

- In the lateral decubitus position, the Veress needle is introduced through a 1.5-cm, ipsilateral hemi-circumferential incision around the umbilicus (Figure 6.2).
- Gas flow can be increased once the correct position of the Veress needle is confirmed and 1 L is insufflated.

DOI: 10.1201/b22928-8

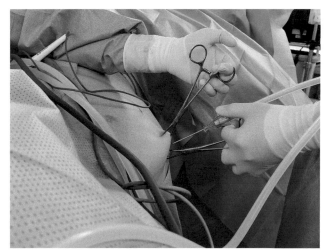

Figure 6.2 Veress needle insertion. The abdomen is stabilized by two towel clips and the needle is perpendicular to the abdomen in 60° position.

Confirmation of correct Veress needle passage and position is explained in Chapter 3, Section 1 "Basic Instrumentation".

- Pneumoperitoneum is created to 15 mmHg for trocar insertion, after which it is set down to 12 mmHg throughout the procedure.

Access can also be obtained with an open (Hasson) technique or under direct vision using an optiview trocar with the laparoscope (Figure 6.3).

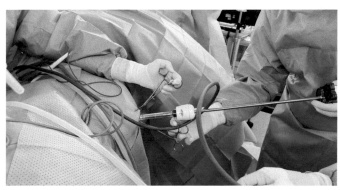

Figure 6.3 Optical trocar insertion. Direct visualization of the abdominal layers by using the scope through a visual obturator.

PORT INSERTION

- An 11-mm trocar is inserted at the access site and a 10-mm, 30° lens laparoscope is introduced to assess:
  - Veress needle and port entry area for any injuries
  - Operation site and kidney outline
  - Presence of adhesion
  - Survey for abnormal anatomy or lesions
  - Entry sites of the next port

- Two 11-mm trocars are inserted, applying the triangulation principle in port placement toward the kidney position (Figure 6.4).

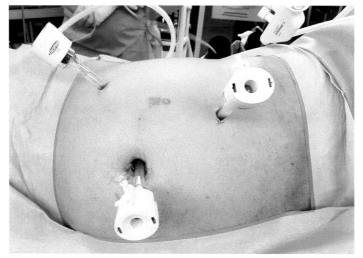

Figure 6.4 Trocar configurations applying the triangulation principle in port placement (for right kidney).

- A fourth trocar of 11 mm is inserted (*at a later step*) opposite to the camera, making a diamond-shaped orientation with other ports.
- For the right kidney, a 5-mm liver retraction trocar is inserted just inferior to the xiphoid process.

> Veress needle and port positions may vary depending on the patient's body habitus, tumor location, kidney anatomy, presence of adhesions and surgeon's preference. However, the principle of triangulation is applied, keeping the instruments at least 7 cm apart.

OPERATING ROOM SETUP AND SURGEON POSITIONS

- The operating room is set up to facilitate a smooth flow of surgery (Figure 6.5).
- The primary surgeon stands at the abdominal side of the patient.
- The first assistant stands caudal to the surgeon, toward the hip, and a second assistant, if needed, stands at the back of the patient.

STEP-BY-STEP SURGERY

ADHESIOLYSIS AND LIVER RETRACTION

- Adhesiolysis is performed if bowel adhesions are present at the operation area or at port entry sites.
- For the right kidney, the liver and gallbladder adhesions are released before introducing the retractor. The right triangular ligament may need to be divided at this step (Figure 6.6).

> To avoid liver injury while inserting the retraction port, a right angle can be applied against the anterior abdominal wall around the entry point of the trocar (Figure 6.7).

- Atraumatic non-crushing locking grasper is introduced and fixed to the diaphragm muscles superior-laterally (Figure 6.8).

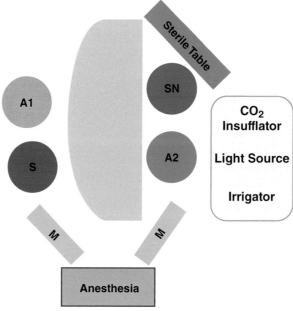

Figure 6.5 Diagram of the operation room setup showing the surgical team positions in relation to the patient, monitors (M) and the accessory machines. *Abbreviations*: GV, gonadal vein; A, assistants; S, primary surgeon; SN, scrub nurse.

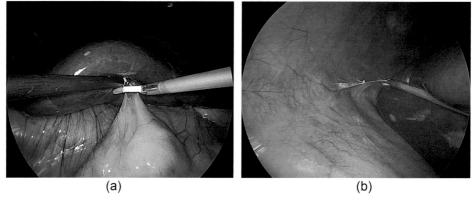

(a)   (b)

Figure 6.6 (a) Releasing the liver from adhesions. (b) Division of the right triangular ligament of the liver.

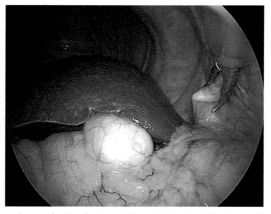

Figure 6.7 Using a right angle against anterior abdominal wall during insertion of the 5-mm liver retraction trocar to avoid liver injury.

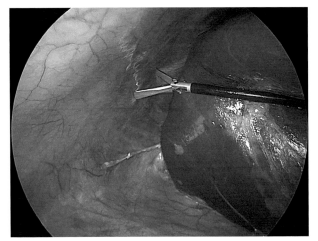

Figure 6.8 Self-retaining liver retraction using a nontraumatic locking grasper.

(DESCENDING OR ASCENDING) COLON MOBILIZATION

- The peritoneum is opened at the white line of Toldt just lateral to the colon, reflecting the bowel medially (Figure 6.9).

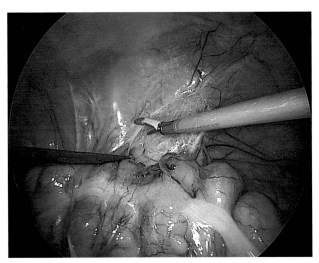

Figure 6.9 The peritoneum is opened at the white line of Toldt. Medial countertraction of the colon is performed by a dissector.

- A plane between the white perinephric fat of Gerota and the yellow fat of the mesocolon is created by blunt and sharp dissection (Figure 6.10).

Meticulous and careful use of an energy device or monopolar scissors at this step is mandatory to avoid injuries to the colon or its mesentery.

- The dissection is carried out from the level of common iliac vessels inferiorly up to the level of the colonic flexure and/or the diaphragm superiorly at the upper pole.

The planes are opened carefully from superficial to deep, layer by layer, up and down along the line of dissection.

Injuries or bleeding in deep and narrow spaces are difficult to manage due to inadequate exposure.

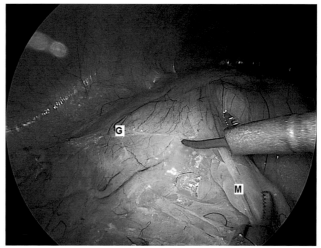

Figure 6.10 Dissection is performed in avascular plane between the white perinephric fat of Gerota (G) and the yellow fat of mesocolon (M).

Dissecting the lateral Gerota attachment at this step must be avoided, as this will drop down the kidney medially and makes the hilar dissection difficult.

Oncologic surgery should be embryologic surgery. If the dissection is performed between the embryologically different planes, it should be easy and oncologically safe. Being an avascular plane, the bleeding should be minimal.

IN THE RIGHT SIDE

- The hepatorenal and posterior coronary ligaments are incised (Figure 6.11).

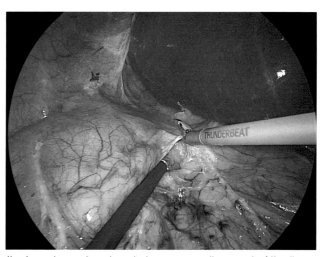

Figure 6.11 Incising the hepatorenal and posterior coronary ligament of the liver.

The division of hepatorenal and posterior coronary ligaments will expose the lateral wall of vena cava above the adrenal gland, duodenum and renal hilum.

- After reflecting the colon medially, the duodenum is identified and Kocherized to reveal the anterior surface of the inferior vena cava (IVC) (Figure 6.12).

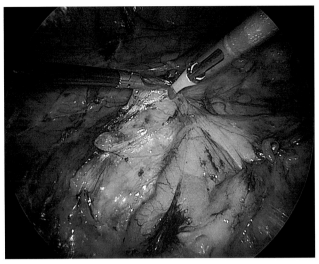

Figure 6.12 Kocherization of the duodenum.

Take care to avoid close contact to the duodenum by cautery or energy device blades.

IN THE LEFT SIDE

- A slightly more extensive colon mobilization is required on the left side to include the splenic flexure, the spleen and the tail of pancreas.
- The incision of splenocolic, linorenal and phrenicocolic ligaments is carefully performed (Figure 6.13).

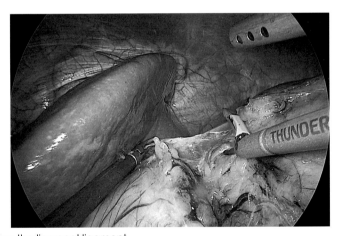

Figure 6.13 Incising the linorenal ligament.

Once the linorenal and spleenocolic ligaments are divided, the spleen, pancreas and colon will drop and be reflected medially. This decreases the risk of injury, during later dissection of the hilum, adrenal gland and upper pole.

Take care to avoid spleen and stomach injury when extensive dissection of the left upper pole attachment is performed.

- The tail of pancreas is further released from the adrenal gland and upper pole of the kidney, taking care to avoid injury to the pancreatic tissue or the splenic vessels (Figure 6.14).

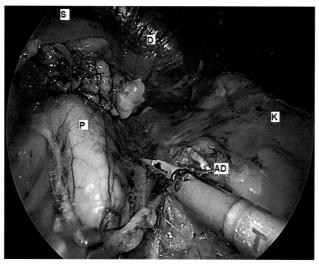

Figure 6.14 Releasing the tail of pancreas (P) further from the adrenal gland (AD) and upper pole kidney (K). The spleen (S) is dropped medially after incising linorenal ligament. *Abbreviation:* D, diaphragm.

PSOAS MUSCLE, URETER AND GONADAL VESSELS

- Inferiorly, the anterior layer of Gerota's fascia is opened and dissected just lateral to IVC in the right side or to the aorta in the left (Figure 6.15).

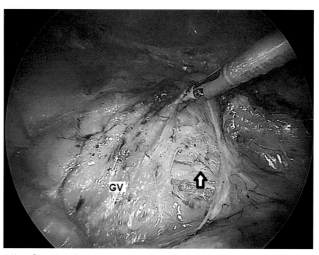

Figure 6.15 Opening the Gerota's fascia. Ureter (arrow) above the psoas muscle (left side). *Abbreviation:* GV, gonadal vein.

- The gonadal vein and ureter are identified in the fibrofatty tissue above the psoas muscle.
- The vein is usually seen first anterior to the ureter.

> In males, if only one tubular structure is identified then it is most likely the vein. To confirm that, it can be followed toward the internal inguinal ring.

- The ureter is clipped below the level of the tumor by size 10 L Hem-o-lok but not divided.
- The gonadal vein can be clipped divided at this step.

Early ligation of the ureter before the kidney manipulation may decrease the chance of tumor cells migration to the bladder.
    On the contrary, delayed ligation after the renal artery is being controlled will decrease the renal blood flow, urine production and ureteric distension.

- At this step, the assistant (fourth) port is inserted opposite to camera, making diamond-shaped configuration with the other ports keeping at least 7-cm in-between (Figure 6.16).

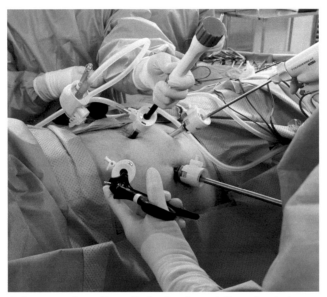

Figure 6.16 Diamond shape configuration with the fourth port (fan retractor).

- A fan retractor is introduced, and the Gerota's fascia with the ureter-gonadal vein packet is retracted anterolaterally, exposing the psoas muscle (Figure 6.17).

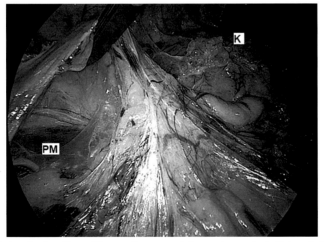

Figure 6.17 Anterolateral retraction of the ureter-gonadal vessels packet. *Abbreviations*: K, kidney; PM, psoas muscle.

> The anterolateral retraction of ureter-gonadal vein packet will stretch the medial and the posterior kidney attachments and will facilitate the dissection.

Take care to avoid excessive traction on the right gonadal vein to prevent avulsion injury at the level of the IVC.

POSTEROMEDIAL DISSECTION

- Once the kidney is on traction, the posterior surface of Gerota will be clearly visualized.
- The posterior areolar attachment of Gerota to the psoas muscle is freed by blunt and sharp dissection (Figure 6.18).

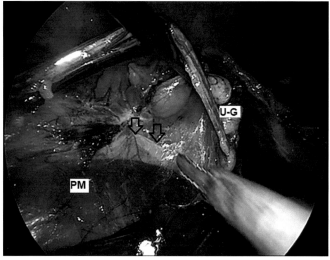

Figure 6.18 Psoas fascia (arrows). *Abbreviations*: PM, psoas muscle; U-G, ureter-gonadal-fatty tissue packet under traction.

Psoas fascia should be released intact to avoid muscle fiber exposure causing unwanted bleeding.

- The anteromedial Gerota attachment is dissected superficially layer by layer to avoid injuries to the gonadal vein or crossing vessels to the kidney and ureter.
- In the right side, the gonadal vein can be seen joining the IVC. It can be clipped and divided to avoid traction injury and significant bleeding (Chapter 5, Figure 5.19).
- The fibro-lymphovascular tissue around the hilum is dissected with caution avoiding inadvertent vascular injuries.
- The bulky tissue attachment or small vessels can be clipped and transected by an energy device.
- Occasionally, hilar or para-aortic lymph nodes are encountered; they are either dissected and excised separately or resected en-bloc with the specimen.

THE PEDICLE

> In the left side, the colon may fall back laterally on the field. It can be retracted to the abdominal wall by a stitch using a suture passer needle (Figure 6.19).

- Once the Gerota attachment around the hilum is cleared, the renal vein can be clearly identified under tension because of traction.

The vena cava in the right and gonadal vein in the left can be used as guiding landmarks to the renal vein.

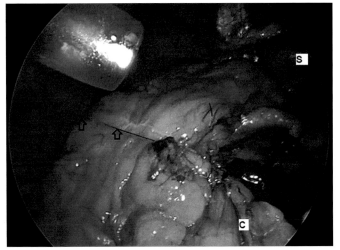

Figure 6.19 Descending colon (C) traction to anterior abdominal wall by PDS thread (arrows). *Abbreviation*: S, spleen.

- The assistant retractor position is adjusted to be just at the lower pole of the kidney giving better exposure with gentle stretch of the pedicle.

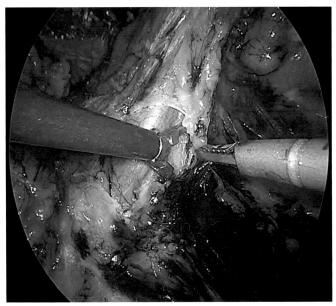

Figure 6.20 Anterior and inferior dissection of the left renal vein.

- The anterior and inferior surfaces of the renal vein are cleared from fibrofatty tissue (Figure 6.20).
- The left gonadal vein may need to be clipped and divided at this level also if interfering with the dissection.
- A lumbar vein joining the left renal vein may be identified. It is isolated, clipped by Hem-o-lok and divided (Figure 6.21).

If the lumbar vein is not well controlled or injured during dissection, it may retract into the muscle and will be hard to catch and control.

Division of the left gonadal and lumbar vein will expose the renal artery.

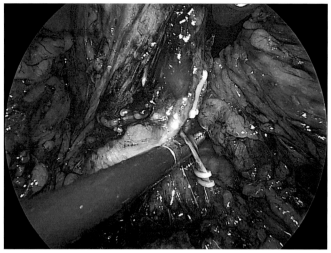

Figure 6.21 Isolation and clip ligation of left lumbar vein.

- The lymphovascular tissue posterior to the renal vein is carefully dissected looking for the renal artery.
- The renal artery is identified by its pulsation or as a white wall tubular structure posterior the vein.

Suction probe can be used to facilitate identifying and dissecting the artery (Figure 6.22).

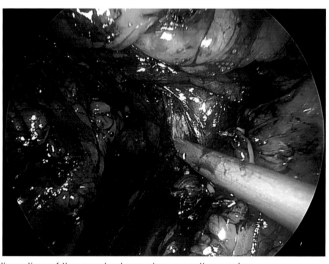

Figure 6.22 Blunt dissection of the renal artery using a suction probe.

- The periarterial tissue is cleared to skeletonize the artery circumferentially using a Maryland or right-angled dissector and energy device (Figure 6.23).
- The tissue bands dissected off the artery are carefully coagulated and divided away from the vessel.

If the renal artery is too deep for clipping, it can be retracted by a vessel loop or carefully grasped by the left-hand Maryland.

If the renal artery needs to be grasped and pulled out, the whole width of the artery should be included between the jaws of the grasper.

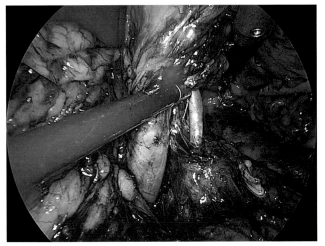

Figure 6.23 Dissection and isolation of the renal artery using left Maryland.

- The artery is clipped proximally by two L-size Hem-o-loks and two metallic titanium ligaclips and divided in-between the ligaclips using straight scissors (Figure 6.24).

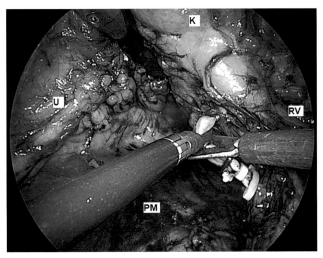

Figure 6.24 Right renal artery is clipped and being divided by straight scissors. Note the arterial wall is completely grasped by Maryland. *Abbreviations*: K, lower pole kidney; PM, psoas muscle; RV, right renal vein; U, ureter.

If there is not enough space for multiple clips at the artery, the renal vein can be dissected and divided first after applying just one clip on the artery.

- Once the artery is clipped and divided, the vein should collapse, if not then look for another artery.

> Reviewing the preoperative imaging study is critical to assess for early branching artery and to rule out multiple or accessory arteries.

In a large and medially displaced left lower pole renal tumor, the superior mesenteric artery may be mistaken with left renal artery.

- The renal vein is dissected and circumferentially freed from the fibrofatty tissue attachment creating an adequate window by a Maryland dissector or a right-angled dissector (Figure 6.25).

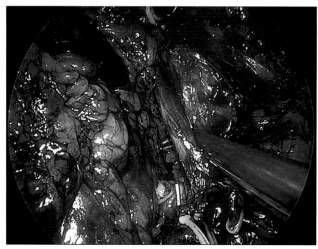

Figure 6.25 Dissection of the renal vein.

The left adrenal vein may be clipped and divided if interfering with dissection or vein ligation.

- A vessel loop is placed around the vein and retracted with a left-hand Maryland (Figure 6.26).
- The renal vein is clipped by two XL-size Hem-o-loks at IVC side and one at kidney side and divided in-between by straight scissors.

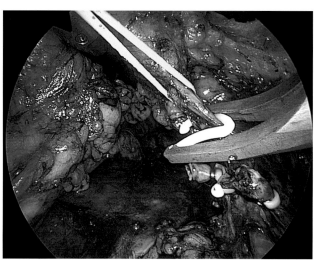

Figure 6.26 The left renal vein is retracted by a vessel loop and clipped using an XL Hem-o-lok. Note that the angle of the clip applicator is oriented to provide a space for next clips and a safe margin for division.

Correct method of clip application is explained in Section 1.

> Using a vessel loop to retract the renal vein will further shrink its wall and facilitate easy control and safe clipping.

ADRENAL GLAND PRESERVATION AND UPPER POLE DISSECTION

- The kidney is dropped down off the retractor and the Gerota's fascia is opened on the kidney just above the divided renal vein.
- The perinephric fat is dissected upward on the anteromedial surface of the kidney (Figure 6.27).

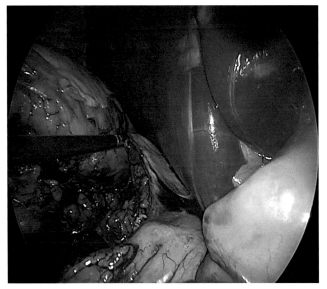

Figure 6.27 Separating the adrenal gland from the upper pole right kidney.

Take care to avoid injuries to aberrant vessels or other structures such as pancreas, IVC and aorta medially.

- After adrenal separation, blunt and sharp dissection using an energy device is continued to free the upper pole.

> To facilitate the left upper pole dissection, wide exposure can be achieved by gentle superior-anterior traction of the spleen by the left-hand Maryland grasper (Figure 6.28).

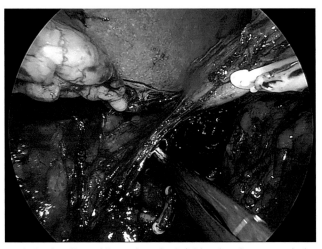

Figure 6.28 Superior-anterior traction of the spleen by left Maryland grasper during the dissection of the left upper pole residual attachment.

ADRENALECTOMY

- Occasionally adrenal gland removal with the kidney is indicated, like in huge upper pole tumor or when adrenal metastasis is suspected on imaging studies.
- On the right side, the extra Gerota dissection begins just lateral to the IVC.

- The adrenal vein is clipped and divided just lateral to its entrance into the IVC.
- On the left side, dissection begins medial to the origin of adrenal vein at the renal vein and just lateral to the aorta.
- The left adrenal vein may not be ligated if the renal vein was proximally divided.

Usually, there are no recognizable or sizable adrenal arteries, and transecting them with an energy device is sufficient.

COMPLETION OF KIDNEY EXCISION

- Starting at the level of the lower pole at inferior Gerota, the kidney is completely freed by blunt and sharp dissection from the lateral abdominal wall.
- The dissection is performed using an energy device through the avascular peritoneal plane between the Gerota's fascia and lateral peritoneal reflection (Figure 6.29).

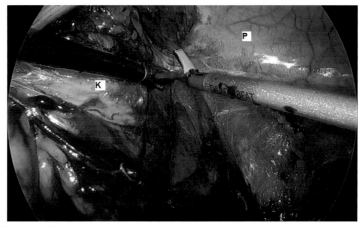

Figure 6.29 Left kidney (K) with Gerota's fascia release from the lateral peritoneal reflection (P).

- The dissection is continued laterally until the upper pole is released off its remaining attachment.
- The kidney is introduced in an endo-catch bag (size depends on the specimen volume).
- The bag is closed and a clip is applied on the thread to ensure the closure.

URETERAL MOBILIZATION

- The ureter is dissected distal to the clip and freed from its peritoneal and fatty-fibrovascular attachment.
- It can be gently grasped by the left-hand Maryland and retracted to facilitate the dissection.

Take care to avoid ureteric violation by rough handling or excessive traction.

- The gonadal vessels crossing anterior to the ureter to enter the internal inguinal ring in males or to the ovaries medially in females can be isolated, clipped and divided (Figure 6.30).

ADDITIONAL PORT INSERTION

- The table is further tilted toward the operation side with a slight Trendelenburg position, and another 11-mm port is added.
- It is inserted contralateral and almost opposite to the distal port, applying the triangulation principle, with the camera at the umbilicus.
- The surgeon's position is exchanged with the assistant's, so the surgeon stands caudal to the assistant and directed to the pelvis.
- The screen location is changed toward the legs to be aligned with the camera, surgeon's vision and operation site.

Principles of surgical setup and trocar configuration are explained in Section 1.

Laparoscopic Radical Nephroureterectomy

84

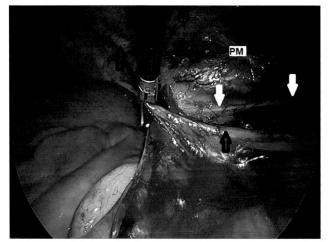

Figure 6.30 Isolation of right gonadal vessels (black arrows). Ureter (white arrows). *Abbreviation:* PM, psoas muscle.

DISTAL URETERIC DISSECTION AND BLADDER CUFF EXCISION

- The peritoneum over the ureter is incised along its course to the bladder (Figure 6.31).

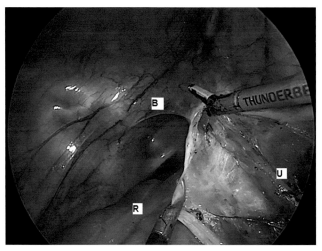

Figure 6.31 Opening the peritoneum along the right ureter (U) toward the bladder (B). *Abbreviation:* R, rectum.

- The ureter is dissected and released from the surrounding attachment using an energy device or monopolar scissor.
- To free the surgeon's left hand, the ureter can be retracted by the assistant using an atraumatic locking grasper and manipulated in different directions to clearly expose the planes of dissection.
- The vas in males (round ligament is females) is seen crossing the ureter anteriorly near the bladder. If interfering with dissection, it can be clipped and divided to enhance ureteric access to the bladder (Figure 6.32).

A branch from the superior vesicle artery is usually identified at the distal ureter and just distal to the crossing vas in males or round ligament in females. It is coagulated or clipped and divided.

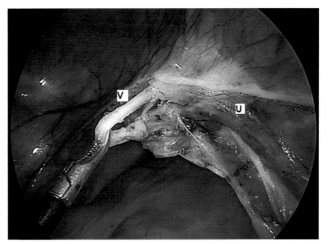

Figure 6.32 Left vas deference (V) crossing anterior to the ureter (U) near the bladder.

- At the ureteric hiatus on the bladder, the periureteric tissue is carefully dissected off the ureter toward bladder wall until the detrusor muscle is seen.
- With the ureter on traction, the bladder mucosa with detrusor muscle fibers will get tented outside (bladder cuff) (Figure 6.33).

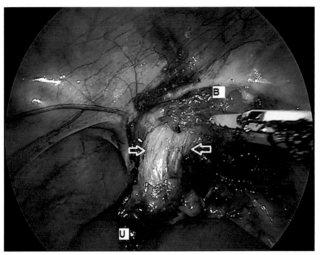

Figure 6.33 Tenting of the bladder mucosa with detrusor muscle fibers (arrows) while the ureter (U) is on traction. *Abbreviation*: B, bladder (left side).

- A 3/0 absorbable V-Loc or PDS stay stitch is placed on the bladder cuff.

A stay stitch at the bladder cuff will prevent bladder wall retraction after transecting the ureter and facilitate the cystostomy closure.

- The ureter is clipped distally by XL-size Hem-o-lok clip and the bladder cuff is transected using monopolar scissors just proximal to the stay stitch (Figure 6.34).
- The ureter is introduced inside the endo-catch bag with the kidney.
- The bladder is closed in one layer by continuous running suturing; using the same stitch, ensure the bladder mucosa is included in the suture line (Figure 6.35).
- The integrity of water-tight closure is assessed by filling the bladder to 150 mL of normal saline observing for leakage.

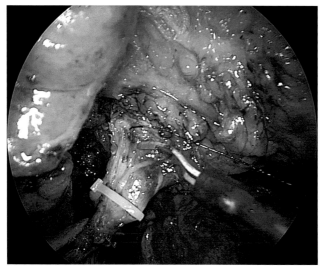

Figure 6.34 Transection of the ureter using monopolar scissors. The ureter is seen clipped and retracted. Note a V-Loc stay stitch on the bladder cuff.

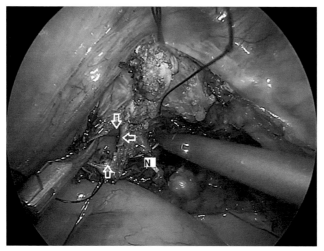

Figure 6.35 Vertical closure of the cystostomy. The needle (N) includes the bladder wall and mucosa (arrows) in the suture line.

DRAIN, SPECIMEN RETRIEVAL AND WOUND CLOSURE

- Drains are inserted and wounds of more than 10 mm are closed using a Carter Thomason suture pass device on 1/0 vicryl stitch.
- The specimen is removed through a muscle splitting Gibson or Pfannenstiel incisions.

A detailed explanation of drain and closure along with figures is provided in Section 1.

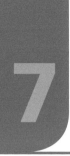

Transperitoneal Laparoscopic Partial Nephrectomy

POSITION

- The patient is positioned in a semi-lateral (60°) decubitus position with the abdomen at the table edge (Figure 7.1).
- Straps, adhesives and supporting pads are applied to stabilize the patient, and the urinary catheter is inserted before the draping.

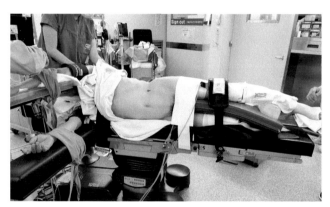

Figure 7.1 Semi-lateral decubitus position. The patient is strapped and supported; shoulder and pressure areas are padded; electrocautery is connected; urethral catheter is inserted; intermittent pneumatic calf compression device and elastic stocking are applied.

> The table is not flexed in a transperitoneal approach to avoid unnecessary rhabdomyolysis and postoperative neuromusculoskeletal pain.
>
> Table flexion may also decrease the working space by pushing the kidney close to the abdominal wall.

ACCESS

- In the lateral decubitus position, Veress needle is introduced through a 1.5-cm ipsilateral hemi-circumferential incision around the umbilicus (Figure 7.2).
- Gas flow can be increased once the Veress needle's correct position is confirmed and 1 L is insufflated.

DOI: 10.1201/b22928-9

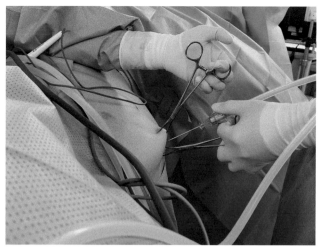

Figure 7.2 Veress needle insertion perpendicular to abdomen in 60° position. The abdominal wall is stabilized by two towel clips.

Confirmation of correct Veress needle passage and position is explained in Chapter 3, Section 1 "Basic Instrumentation".

- Pneumoperitoneum is created to at least 15 mmHg for trocar insertion, after which it is set down to 12 mmHg throughout the procedure.

Access can also be obtained using the open (Hasson) technique or by direct vision using an optiview trocar with the laparoscope (Chapter 5, Figure 5.3).

> For the left side, as more lateral bowel dissection is required to expose the renal hilum, a closed or open access (Hasson) can be obtained at the ipsilateral pararectus muscle just distal to the umbilicus.

PORT INSERTION

- An 11-mm trocar is inserted at the access site and a 10-mm, 30° lens laparoscope is introduced to assess:

  - Veress needle and port entry area for any injuries
  - Operation site and kidney outline
  - Presence of adhesions
  - Survey for abnormal anatomy or lesions
  - Entry sites of the next port

- If the open access wound obtained is quiet large for the 11-mm trocar, then a blunt tip balloon trocar with a sponge collar is used to secure the port and minimize air leakage (Figure 7.3).
- Two 12-mm trocars are inserted applying the triangulation principle in port placement toward the kidney position (Figure 7.4).
- A fourth trocar of 11 mm is inserted (*at a later step*) opposite to the camera, making a diamond-shaped orientation with other ports.
- For the right kidney, a 5-mm liver retraction trocar is inserted just inferior to the xiphoid process.

> Access site and port positions may vary depending on the patient's body habitus, tumor location, kidney anatomy, presence of adhesions and surgeon's preference. The principle of triangulation is applied, keeping the instruments at least 7 cm apart.

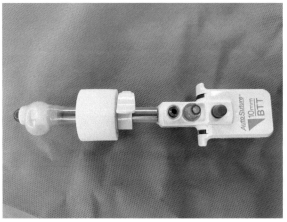

Figure 7.3 Blunt tip balloon trocar with foam sponge collar.

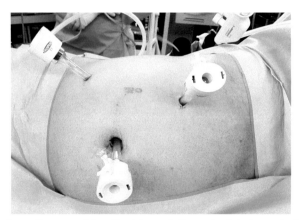

Figure 7.4 Trocar configurations applying the triangulation principle in port placement (for right kidney).

OPERATION ROOM SETUP AND SURGEON POSITIONS

- The operating room is set up to facilitate a smooth flow of surgery (Figure 7.5).
- The surgeon stands at the abdominal side of the patient.
- The first assistant stands caudal to the surgeon, toward the hip, and a second assistant, if needed, stands at the back of the patient.

STEP-BY-STEP SURGERY

ADHESIOLYSIS AND LIVER RETRACTION

- Adhesiolysis is performed if bowel adhesions are present at the operation area or at port entry sites.
- For the right kidney, the liver and gallbladder adhesions are released before introducing the retractor.
  - The triangular ligament may need to be divided at this step (Figure 7.6).
- The liver retraction trocar is inserted just inferior to xiphoid process.

To avoid liver injury while inserting the retraction port, a right-angled grasper can be applied against the anterior abdominal wall around the entry point of the trocar (Figure 7.7).

- Atraumatic, non-crushing locking grasper is introduced and fixed to the diaphragm muscles supero-laterally (Figure 7.8).

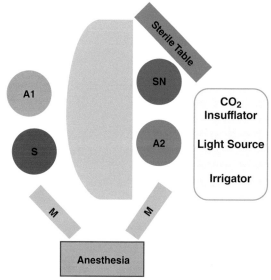

Figure 7.5 Diagram of the operation room setup showing the surgical team positions in relation to the patient, monitors (M) and the accessory machines. *Abbreviations*: A1, first assistant; A2, second assistant; S, primary surgeon; SN, scrub nurse.

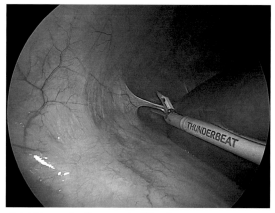

Figure 7.6 Division of the right triangular ligament of the liver.

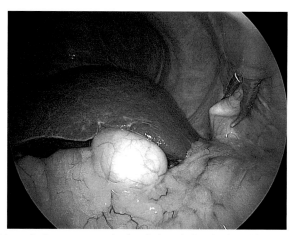

Figure 7.7 Using a right-angled grasper against anterior abdominal wall to avoid liver injury during insertion of the 5-mm liver retraction trocar.

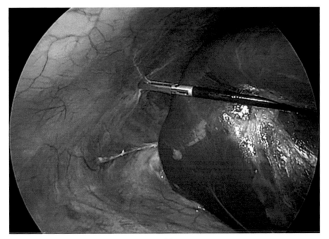

Figure 7.8 Liver retraction using a non-crushing locking grasper.

COLON (DESCENDING OR ASCENDING) MOBILIZATION

- The peritoneum is opened at the white line of Toldt just lateral to the colon, reflecting the bowel medially (Figure 7.9).

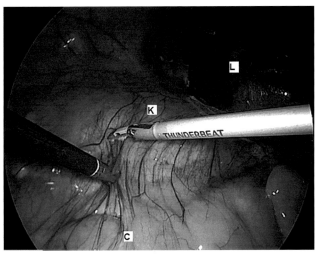

Figure 7.9 The peritoneum is opened at the white line of Toldt. *Abbreviations*: C, ascending colon; L, liver on traction; K, right kidney covered by peritoneum.

- A plane between the white perinephric fat of Gerota and the yellow fat of the mesocolon is created by blunt and sharp dissection (Figure 7.10).

Meticulous and careful use of energy device or monopolar scissors at this step is mandatory to avoid injuries to the colon or its mesentery.

- The dissection is carried out from the level of common iliac vessels inferiorly up to the level of the colonic flexure and the diaphragm superiorly at the upper pole.

The planes are carefully opened from superficial to deep, layer by layer, up and down along the line of dissection.

Injuries or bleeding in deep and narrow spaces are difficult to manage due to inadequate exposure.

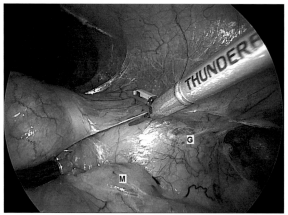

Figure 7.10 Dissection through avascular plane between the white perinephric fat of Gerota (G) and the yellow fat of mesocolon (M).

Dissecting the lateral Gerota attachment at this step must be avoided. That will drop down the kidney medially and make the hilar dissection difficult.

Oncologic surgery should be embryologic surgery. If the dissection is performed between the embryologically different planes, it should be easy and oncologically safe. Being an avascular plane, the bleeding should be minimal.

IN THE RIGHT SIDE

- The hepatorenal and posterior coronary ligaments of the liver are incised and extended to the diaphragm if complete kidney mobilization is required (Figure 7.11).

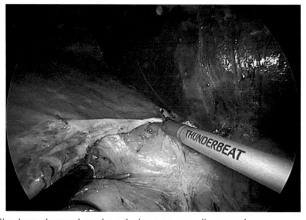

Figure 7.11 Incising the hepatorenal and posterior coronary ligaments.

The division of hepatorenal and posterior coronary ligaments will expose the lateral wall of vena cava above the adrenal gland, duodenum and renal hilum (Figure 7.12).

- After reflecting the colon medially, the duodenum is identified and Kocherized to reveal the anterior surface of the inferior vena cava (IVC) (Figure 7.13).

Close contact to the duodenum by cautery or energy device blades must be avoided.

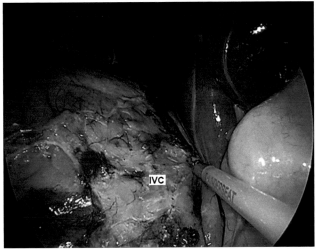

Figure 7.12 Infrahepatic IVC and upper surface of right renal vein can be visualized after incising the hepatorenal and coronary ligaments.

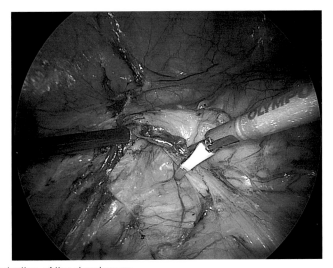

Figure 7.13 Kocherization of the duodenum.

IN THE LEFT SIDE

- The usual extensive colon mobilization and upper pole dissection may not be necessary in partial nephrectomy unless complete mobilization of the kidney is required depending on tumor size and location.
- The splenocolic, linorenal and phrenicocolic ligaments are carefully incised (Figure 7.14).

> Once these ligaments are divided, the spleen, pancreas and colon will drop and reflect medially. This decreases the risk of organ injury, during later dissection of the hilum, adrenal gland and upper pole.

Take care to avoid spleen and stomach injury if extensive dissection of the left upper pole attachment is performed.

- The tail of pancreas is further released from the adrenal gland and upper pole of the kidney, taking care to avoid injury to the pancreatic tissue or the splenic vessels (Figure 7.15).

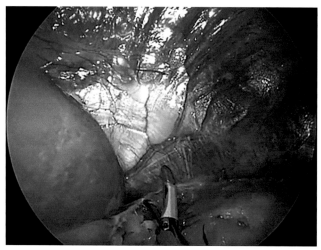

Figure 7.14 Incising the linorenal ligament.

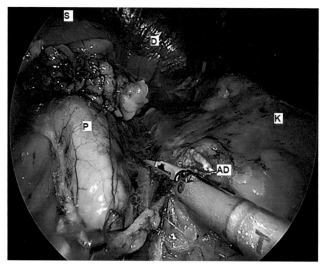

Figure 7.15 Releasing the tail of pancreas (P) from the Gerota-containing adrenal gland (AD) and upper pole kidney (K). *Abbreviations*: D, diaphragm; S, dropped spleen.

PSOAS MUSCLE, URETER AND GONADAL VESSELS

Ureteric and gonadal dissection and isolation may not be necessary unless kidney mobilization is required or in case of lower pole tumor.

- Inferiorly, the anterior layer of Gerota's fascia is opened and dissected just lateral to IVC in the right side or to aorta in the left (Figure 7.16).
- The gonadal vein and ureter are identified in the fibrofatty tissue above the psoas muscle.
- They are dissected together with surrounding fat and released from the psoas muscle.
- The assistant (fourth) port is inserted opposite to the camera, making a diamond-shaped configuration with the other ports, keeping at least 7 cm in-between (Figure 7.17).
- A retractor is introduced and the Gerota's fascia with the ureter-gonadal vein packet is retracted anterolaterally exposing the psoas muscle.

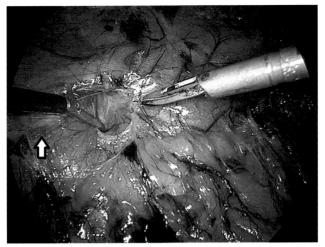

Figure 7.16 Opening the Gerota's fascia to reveal the ureter and gonadal vessels (arrow) above the psoas muscle.

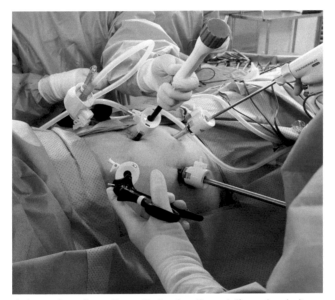

Figure 7.17 Diamond-shaped configuration with the fourth port (fan retractor).

> The anterolateral retraction of ureter-gonadal vein packet will stretch the medial and the posterior Gerota attachment and facilitate the dissection (Figure 7.18).

Take care to avoid excessive traction to prevent renal arterial spasm or right gonadal vein avulsion injury at the level of the IVC.

POSTEROMEDIAL DISSECTION

- Once the kidney is on traction, the posterior surface of Gerota's fascia will be clearly visualized.
- The posterior areolar attachment of Gerota to the psoas muscle is freed by blunt and sharp dissection.

Psoas fascia should be released intact to avoid muscle fibers exposure and unwanted bleeding.

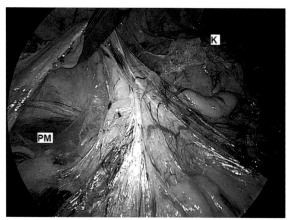

Figure 7.18 Anterolateral retraction of the ureter-gonadal vessels packet. Anteromedial attachment is stretched for easy and safe dissection. *Abbreviations*: K, kidney; PM, psoas muscle.

- The anteromedial Gerota attachment is dissected superficially layer by layer to avoid injuries to the gonadal vein or crossing vessels to the kidney and ureter.
- In the right side, the gonadal vein may be seen joining the IVC. It can be clipped and divided to avoid traction injury and significant bleeding (Figure 7.19).

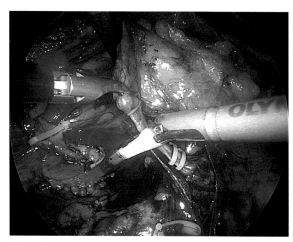

Figure 7.19 Right gonadal vein.

- Fibro-lymphovascular tissue at the hilum around the pedicle is dissected superficially and with caution avoiding inadvertent vascular injuries.
- The bulky tissue attachment or small vascular branches can be clipped and/or transected by monopolar scissors.

> Applying multiple clips around the pedicle should be avoided. They may interfere with vascular clamping, particularly in case of emergency.

THE PEDICLE

> In the left side, the colon may fall back laterally on the field; it can be retracted by a stitch using a suture passer needle through the abdominal wall (Figure 7.20).

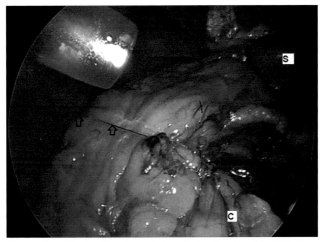

Figure 7.20 Descending colon (C) traction to anterior abdominal wall by PDS thread (arrows).
Abbreviation: S, spleen.

- Once the medial Gerota's attachment around the hilum is cleared, the renal vein can be clearly identified under mild tension because of gentle traction.

The vena cava in the right and gonadal vein in the left can be used as guidance landmarks to the renal vein.

> If complete kidney mobilization is not indicated, then the pedicle can be approached directly through the hilum without extensive inferior or superior dissection.

- The assistant retractor position is adjusted to be just at the lower pole of the kidney giving better exposure with gentle stretch of the pedicle.
- The anterior and inferior surfaces of the renal vein are cleared from fibrofatty tissue.
- The left gonadal vein may need to be clipped at this level if interfering with dissection.
- A lumbar vein joining the left renal vein may be identified. It is isolated, clipped by Hem-o-lok and divided (Figure 7.21).

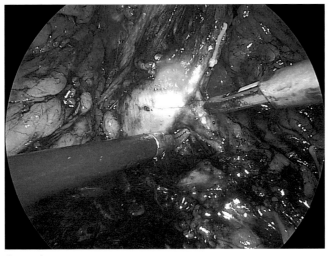

Figure 7.21 Left lumbar vein.

If the lumbar vein is not well controlled or is injured during dissection, it may retract into the muscle and will be hard to catch and control.

> Division of the left gonadal and lumbar vein will expose the renal artery.

- The tissue posterior to the renal vein is carefully dissected looking for the renal artery which can be identified by its pulsation or as a white tubular structure (Figure 7.22).

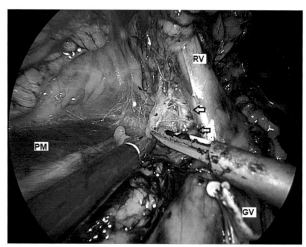

Figure 7.22 Perivascular tissue dissection using Maryland dissector and ultrasonic shear. *Abbreviations*: Arrows, renal artery; GV, clipped right gonadal vein; PM, psoas muscle; RV, renal vein.

- The tissue bands dissected off the artery are carefully coagulated and divided away from the vessel using a left Maryland and right-hand ultrasonic shear.

> Suction probe can be used to facilitate identifying and dissecting the artery.

The artery is circumferentially freed and a wide window is created.

Complete arterial skeletonization from the perivascular adventitia is not necessary.

- The artery is encircled by a vessel loop, and a Hem-o-lok clip is applied on the loop (Figure 7.23).

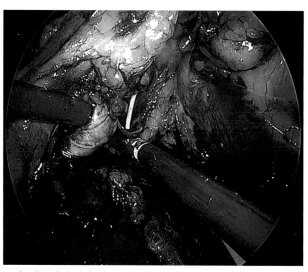

Figure 7.23 The left renal artery is isolated on a vessel loop.

Laparoscopic Partial Nephrectomy

> To avoid excessive bleeding surprise during resection, reviewing the preoperative imaging study to assess for early branching artery and to rule out multiple or accessory arteries is crucial.

- If required, the vein can be further dissected from the fibrofatty tissue and circumferentially freed, creating an adequate window.
- A vessel loop is placed around the vein and the loop is clipped.
- The artery and vein can be isolated both together on a vessel loop if the pedicle dissection is difficult or in case a laparoscopic Satinsky single clamping was planned (Figure 7.24).

> The vessel loop is utilized to manipulate the vessel for accurate clamping. It also provides an easy, safe and fast approach in case of emergency or severe bleeding.

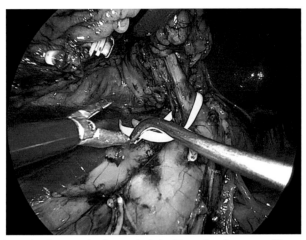

Figure 7.24 Both right renal artery and vein are isolated together in a vessel loop.

ADRENAL GLAND SEPARATION

- In case of upper pole tumor, or when whole kidney mobilization is required, the adrenal gland is dissected and separated from the kidney.
- The Gerota's fascia is opened just above the renal vein and the perinephric fat is dissected upward immediately on the anteromedial surface of renal parenchyma.
- The adrenal gland is separated from the upper pole of the kidney by blunt and sharp dissection using electrocautery or energy device.

Take care to avoid injuries to aberrant vessels to the upper pole or structures such as pancreas, IVC and aorta medially.

TUMOR DISSECTION

> For precise tumor resection and to avoid positive margins, excessive bleeding or long ischemia time, it is crucial for the tumor to be circumferentially accessible.

- Once the tumor area is localized, with or without kidney mobilization, the Gerota's fascia is opened near the tumor location on the normal parenchyma.
- The perinephric fat is cleared off the parenchyma at least 1 cm beyond the tumor edge.
- If possible, it is better not to remove the fat covering the tumor as it can be used to grasp and manipulate the mass during dissection.

If the tumor is endophytic or its limit is undetermined, an intraoperative ultrasound can be utilized to delineate the mass.

PEDICLE CLAMPING

- Once tumor area is prepared and kidney position is adjusted for easy access around the tumor, frusemide and mannitol can be given 15 minutes before pedicle clamping as reno-protectant.
- The line of resection is marked by cautery on the normal parenchyma capsule keeping about 5 mm of safe margin around the tumor (Figure 7.25).

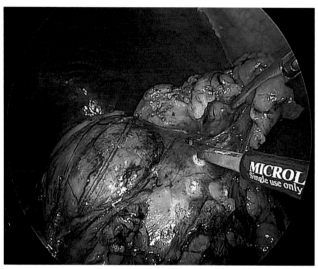

Figure 7.25 The perinephric fat is dissected off the renal capsule, 1 cm beyond the tumor margins, and resection line is marked by cautery. Note the kidney stabilization by the assistant locking grasper.

> To provide further kidney stabilization to achieve an optimal angle for easy tumor resection and renorrhaphy, the Gerota's fascia can be retracted to the abdominal wall by a PDS stitch using a suture pass needle (Figure 7.26).

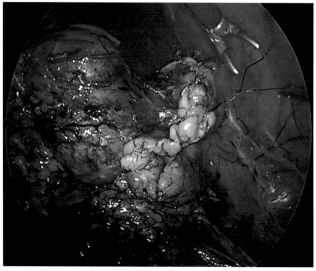

Figure 7.26 Kidney stabilization by PDS stitch using a suture pass needle.

- The artery is retracted by the vessel loop to open a safe window for the Bulldog vascular clamp (Figure 7.27).

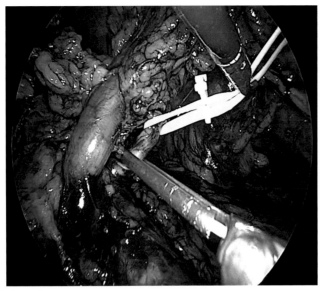

Figure 7.27 Pedicel clamping.

Take care to be steady when introducing the Bulldog clamp to avoid poking the vessels or going further inside blindly.

- The warm ischemia time is set once the artery is clamped.

If the main artery is clamped, the vein should collapse, if not then look for another artery.

> Clamping the vein is usually not necessary unless the tumor is large or central or has got a sizable vein seen on preoperative images. This may provide a bloodless field during tumor resection and renorrhaphy.

TUMOR RESECTION

- The marked parenchyma around the tumor is incised circumferentially and superficially using cold scissors (Figure 7.28).
- The curve of the scissors is directed downward and away from the tumor to facilitate the resection of the tumor to accurate depth and width.

Using electrocautery or energy device for resection may obscure the demarcation of normal tumor tissue and can alter the histological structure.

- The tumor violation during resection must be avoided, and the resection line exposure can be achieved by manipulating the tumor fat or by gentle back traction using the other hand instrument.
- The assistant should apply a reasonable parenchymal pressure in addition to continuous suction-irrigation of blood to improve the vision.

> Irrigation is preferred over suction to clear the field of vision, as excessive suction reduces the intraperitoneal pressure causing bothersome back bleeding.

Keeping a gauze piece in the field for hemostasis may be necessary if significant bleeding is anticipated.

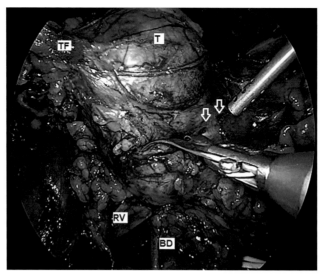

Figure 7.28 Tumor (T) is resected at the marked parenchyma (arrows) directing the scissors downward. The mass is retracted by its fat (TF) using the left-hand grasper. *Abbreviations*: BD, Bulldog vascular clamp; RV, renal vein.

- The incision is deepened by sharp and blunt dissection all around toward the base of tumor (Figure 7.29).

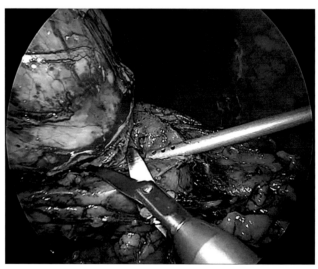

Figure 7.29 Resection of the tumor base. The assistant applies a gentle countertraction on the renal parenchyma and provides suction/irrigation during resection.

- Once the deepest portion of the tumor is incised, the scissors curve is directed upward.

> Reviewing the preoperative images to evaluate the tumor size, depth and configuration is crucial.

Active arterial bleeder during or after tumor resection can be clipped by a small size clip.

- Once the tumor is completely excised, it is placed into an endo-catch bag which is closed, secured by Hem-o-lok and left aside.

RENAL RECONSTRUCTION

- The resection bed is oversewn using a 23-cm, 3/0 V-Loc absorbable stitch on 1/2 circle of (26mm) V-20 needle.
- The stitch is inserted through the renal capsule at the distal end of the wound.

> An anchoring Hem-o-lok clip at the tail end of the stitch will ensure a tense suturing without cutting through the parenchyma (Figure 7.30).

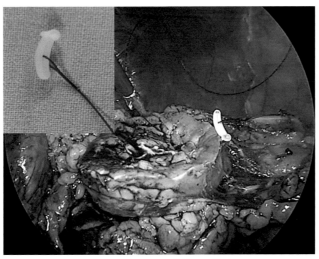

Figure 7.30 An anchoring Hem-o-lok clip at the end of V-Loc stitch.

- The needle is introduced just deep enough to include part of the cortex, medulla and pelvicalyceal system together in a continuous running suturing (Figure 7.31).

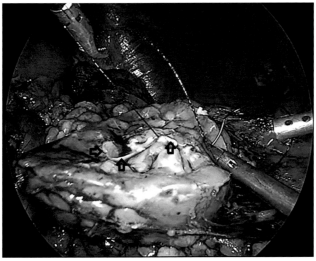

Figure 7.31 Renal reconstruction using a V-Loc stitch includes the renal parenchyma, blood vessels and pelvicalyceal system. Opened calyces are shown by arrows.

- At the stitch exit of the wound, a clip is applied on the renal capsule, maximizing the tension of the suture line (Figure 7.32).

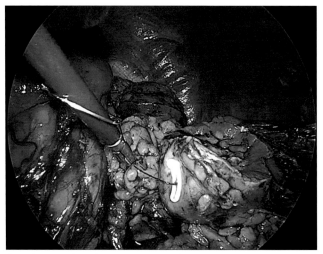

Figure 7.32 The renal bed reconstruction suture line is tightened by applying a clip at the V-Loc stitch exit on the renal capsule.

- If the resection area is large, then two or more stitches are used, dividing the bed into two or more parts.

Careful renal tissue handling and slow meticulous suturing are mandatory to avoid tissue laceration or bleeding, leading to a long ischemia time.

- The Bulldog clamps are carefully removed, making sure that the jaws are opened well enough to avoid significant injuries, and resection area is inspected for active bleeding.

Vein clamp is removed before the arterial one.

> Early pedicle unclamping approach will reduce the ischemia time and facilitate identifying active bleeding for better control.

- A second layer renorrhaphy is performed using a 33-cm, 3/0 PDS stitch on 1/2 circle (31 mm) MH-1 needle.
- The renal defect is closed by approximating the parenchyma over the tumor bed (Figure 7.33).

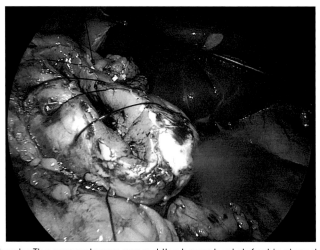

Figure 7.33 Renorrhaphy. The parenchyma around the tumor bed defect is closed by PDS stitch.

In hilar masses, the tumor bed reconstruction is carefully performed to avoid vascular ligation or injuries, and renorrhaphy may not always be possible.

- If the resection bed is bleeding, the renorrhaphy parenchymal reconstruction is performed over a hemostatic agent such as TachoSil and/or surgical (Figure 7.34).

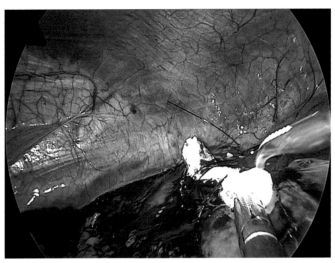

Figure 7.34 Renorrhaphy over a TachoSil roll.

- The suture lines are tightened by placing Hem-o-lok clips at each side of the stitches on the renal capsule (Figure 7.35).

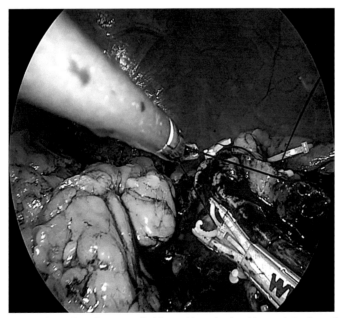

Figure 7.35 The renorrhaphy suture lines are tightened by placing Hem-o-lok clips at each side of the stitches on the renal capsule.

- A hemostatic agent or perinephric fat can be utilized to cover the suture line or residual gap if present.

A second layer renorrhaphy may not be necessary if there is no significant bleeding or urine leak after renal pedicle unclamping, particularly in small defects.

Tumor bed suturing and application of the hemostatic agent such as tissue glue or Surgicel should be adequate.

- If the kidney was completely mobilized, then nephropexy is performed. The Gerota's fascia is clipped to the lateral peritoneal reflection on the lateral abdominal wall by Hem-o-lok clips (Figure 7.36).

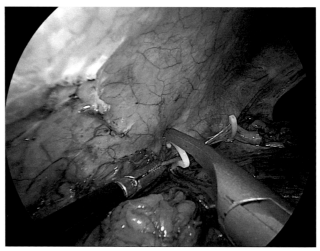

Figure 7.36 Nephropexy.

SPECIMEN RETRIEVAL, DRAIN INSERTION AND WOUND CLOSURE

- The specimen is removed through the access port site or through a Gibson incision if large.
- A drain is inserted and the fascia of wounds more the 10 mm are closed by using Carter Thomason needle pass device on 1/0 vicryl stitch.

The detailed explanation of drain and closure along with figures is provided in Section 1.

8 Retroperitoneal Laparoscopic Simple Nephrectomy

POSITION

- The patient is positioned in a complete lateral decubitus (90°) position with the back at the table edge.
- Table is flexed at the level of the umbilicus (Figure 8.1).

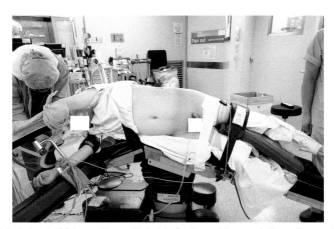

Figure 8.1 Complete lateral (90°) position with table flexion at the umbilicus. The patient is strapped and supported; shoulder and pressure areas are padded; electrocautery is connected; urethral catheter is inserted; intermittent pneumatic calf compression device and elastic stocking are applied.

- Straps, adhesives and supporting pads are applied to stabilize the patient, and the urinary catheter is inserted before the draping.

Flexing the table at a complete lateral decubitus position increases the working space by increasing the distance between the costal margin and iliac crest and the distance between the quadratus lumborum and colon.

ACCESS AND FIRST TROCAR INSERTION

- Access is achieved by open technique in the lateral position.
- A 2-cm incision, 2 cm superior and medial to anterior superior iliac spine (ASIS), is made (Figure 8.2).
- The wound is deepened by muscle splitting using a straight hemostat directing it perpendicular to the patient axis until the retroperitoneal fat is seen.

DOI: 10.1201/b22928-10

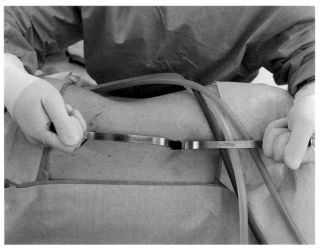

Figure 8.2 Retroperitoneal access. A 2-cm wound 2 cm superior and medial to the ASIS. Fascial layers are exposed by S retractors.

The wound layer exposure and separation is achieved by S retractors and the aid of laparoscopic bright light if required.

- A wet index finger is introduced into the retroperitoneum and a space is created.
- Finger dissection is performed by gentle sweeping movement between the psoas muscle posteriorly and the Gerota's fascia and peritoneal reflection anteriorly.

> To prevent peritoneal injury while accessing the retroperitoneal space, directing the hemostat or finger dissection anteromedially must be avoided.

- Once a maximum space is achieved by finger dissection, a balloon dilator is inserted parallel to psoas muscle and directed cranially (Figure 8.3).

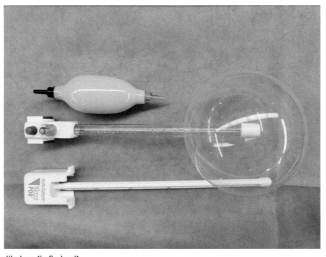

Figure 8.3 Balloon dilator (inflated).

- The balloon is inflated by around 400 mL of air (35–40 pumps), and an obvious tense distension is observed.
- Balloon dilatation can also be performed under a direct laparoscopic vision.

Keeping the balloon inflated for a couple of minutes may provide a local retroperitoneal hemostasis.

- A blunt tip balloon trocar with a sponge collar is introduced to secure the port and minimize the leakage (Figure 8.4).

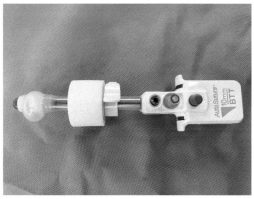

Figure 8.4 Blunt tip balloon trocar with foam sponge collar.

- Gas is insufflated through this port and pneumoretroperitoneum is created to minimum of 12 mmHg.
- A 10-mm laparoscope of 30° lens is introduced to assess:

  - Active bleeding from the access or balloon dissection
  - Peritoneal injuries
  - Gerota's fascia with kidney and psoas muscle outline
  - The entry sites of next trocars

OTHER TROCAR INSERTIONS

- Two working ports are inserted under vision at or just cephalic to the midway between the costal margin and iliac crest (Figure 8.5):

  - An 11-mm port at the anterior axillary line.
  - An 11-mm port at the posterior axillary line.

- An assistant port of 11 mm (if required) for retraction is inserted at the mid-axillary line just below the costal margin.

The access and port sites may differ depending on the kidney anatomy and surgeon's preference.

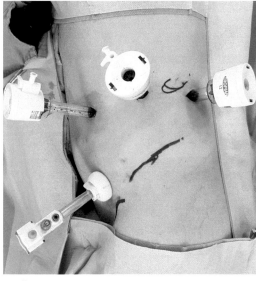

Figure 8.5 The port configurations.

To ensure a safe trocar entry, the posterolateral fat and the anteromedial peritoneum can be dissected off the abdominal wall using a suction probe or monopolar scissors.

OPERATING ROOM SETUP AND SURGEON POSITIONS

- The operation table is lowered to the maximum.
- The surgeon stands at the back of the patient while the assistant stands at the abdominal side.
- The screens are placed toward the patient head (Figure 8.6).

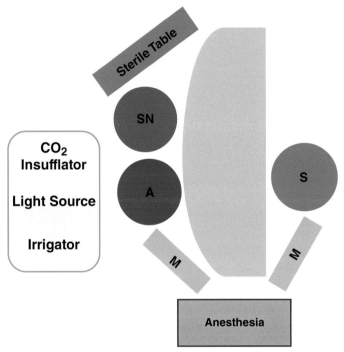

Figure 8.6 Diagram of the operation room setup showing the surgical team positions in relation to the patient, monitors (M) and the accessory machines. *Abbreviations*: A, assistant surgeon; S, surgeon; SN, scrub nurse.

STEP-BY-STEP SURGERY

GEROTA'S FASCIA AND PSOAS MUSCLE DISSECTION

- The paranephric fat is dissected off the Gerota's fascia and psoas muscle (Figure 8.7).

The narrow working space and the anatomic limitations with no clear landmarks are the main challenges of the retroperitoneal approach.

The psoas muscle is the key orientation and should always be in a longitudinal horizontal view.

- Careful and meticulous dissection is continued on the psoas muscle toward the kidney without violating the psoas fascia.
- The Gerota's fascia is incised posteromedially as far as possible to avoid injuring the peritoneum, and the incision is extended parallel to the psoas muscle (Figure 8.8).

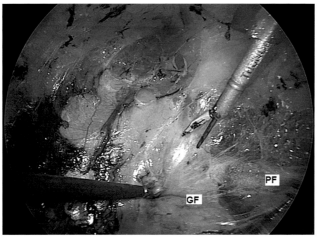

Figure 8.7 Gerota fascia (GF) and psoas fascia (PF).

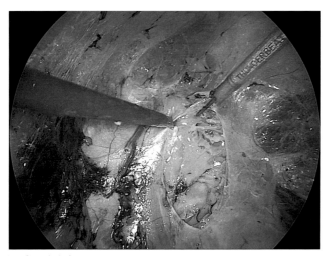

Figure 8.8 Incising the Gerota's fascia.

In case of radical nephrectomy, the dissection is carried out in the avascular plane between the psoas and Gerota's fascia.

- The perinephric fat is dissected toward the hilum aiming for the pedicle.
- If traction is required, an assistant port can be inserted at this step through the anterior axillary line just below the costal margin.
- Retracting the kidney anteromedially by the assistant will further expose the dissection plane and keep the hilum stretched (Figure 8.9).

Keeping the kidney suspended to peritoneum by avoiding anterior dissection early during surgery will prevent it from falling on the hilum.

Dissecting deep medially may injure the vena cava, duodenum on the right side, or the aorta and superior mesenteric artery on the left.

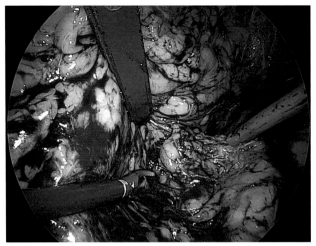

Figure 8.9 Renal hilum dissection. Exposure achieved by fan retractor (FR). Keeping the psoas muscle in view is important for anatomical orientation.

- If difficulty is encountered finding the pedicle, the dissection is carried out inferiorly looking for the lower pole and ureter which is then followed until the hilum.
- The ureter can be identified as a longitudinal white tubular structure with peristalsis parallel to the psoas muscle.

THE PEDICLE

Camera anatomical orientation when dealing with the pedicle is critical to avoid mistaking the renal vessels with other vessels or vital structures.

- At the hilum, the renal artery can be recognized by its pulsation over the fat or seen as a vertically oriented white tubular structure.
- The renal artery is dissected from its periarterial neurolymphatic tissue using a Maryland, suction probe and energy device (Figure 8.10).

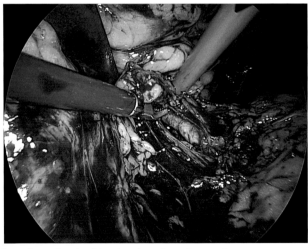

Figure 8.10 Renal artery dissection by Maryland and suction probe.

- In the left side, the lumbar vein can be encountered medially, before the renal artery, and just lateral to the aorta. It can be clipped using Hem-o-lok clips and divided in-between.
- The artery is circumferentially isolated and a wide window around it is created.
- It is clipped proximally by two L-size Hem-o-loks and two metallic titanium ligaclips and divided in-between the ligaclips using straight scissors (Figure 8.11).

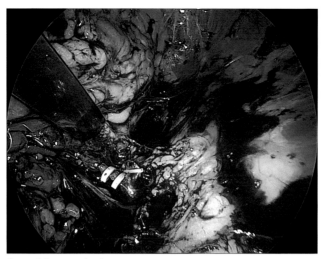

Figure 8.11 Clip ligation of the renal artery.

Reviewing the preoperative imaging study is crucial to assess for early branching artery and to rule out multiple or accessory arteries.

- The renal vein is usually seen anterior and inferior to the artery. It is dissected and circumferentially isolated.
- The perivascular connective tissue is dissected off the vessels with a left-hand Maryland. The tissue is cauterized and divided by an energy device away from the vessel (Figure 8.12).

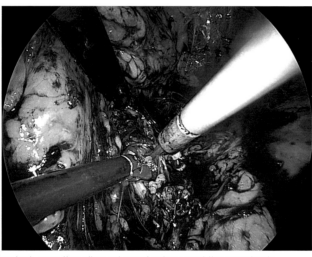

Figure 8.12 Dissection between the clipped renal artery and the renal vein.

- On the left side, the adrenal and gonadal vein may be clipped and divided if interfering with renal vein dissection.
- The renal vein is clipped by two XL-size Hem-o-lok clips at inferior vena cava (IVC) side and one clip at the kidney side and divided in-between by straight scissors (Figure 8.13).

In case of a large renal vein, a vessel loop is placed around the vein and retracted with a left-hand Maryland so it collapses and shrinks for easy clipping.

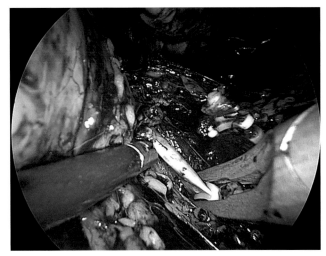

Figure 8.13 Clip ligation of the renal vein.

COMPLETION OF KIDNEY DISSECTION AND LIGATION OF THE URETER

- The kidney is released off its posterior attachment until the upper pole (Figure 8.14).

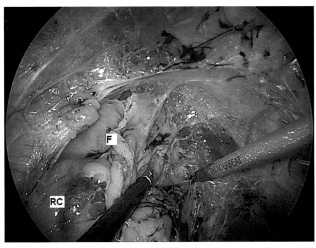

Figure 8.14 Releasing the posterolateral attachment of the upper pole. *Abbreviations*: F, perinephric fat; RC, renal cyst.

- Anteriorly, the kidney is freed from the peritoneum by meticulous blunt and sharp dissection with minimal use of cautery to prevent peritoneal injury (Figure 8.15).

If the peritoneum is perforated, the gas will leak to the peritoneal cavity and may compromise the retroperitoneal space. There are three ways to overcome this situation:

1. Suturing or clipping of the peritoneal gap.
2. Retraction with fan retractor through an additional trocar to minimize the leak.
3. Enlarge the peritoneal incision.

Take care to avoid injuries to the IVC and duodenum in the right side and the spleen, tail of pancreas and aorta in the left side.

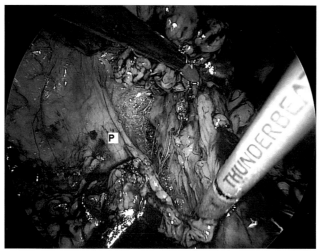

Figure 8.15 Anterior dissection through avascular plane between the peritoneum (P) and Gerota's fascia with perinephric fat.

- During inferior Gerota dissection, the ureter is identified, clipped and divided, if this was not performed at initial steps.

ADRENAL GLAND PRESERVATION AND UPPER POLE DISSECTION

- The perinephric fat is dissected upward on the anteromedial surface of the kidney parenchyma just superior to the divided pedicle (Figure 8.16).

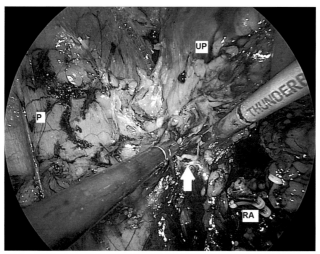

Figure 8.16 Dissection of the adrenal gland (arrow). *Abbreviations*: P, peritoneum; RA, clipped renal artery stump; UP, upper pole of the kidney.

The fatty layers are dissected superficially to avoid injuries to any aberrant vessels of the upper pole.

- Once the adrenal gland is separated, the upper pole is freed from the residual attachment.

SPECIMEN RETRIEVAL, DRAIN INSERTION AND WOUND CLOSURE

- The kidney is introduced in an endo-catch bag.
- The hemostasis is assessed and a drain is inserted if indicated.
- The specimen is removed through extended camera port (access) site and the wound is closed in layers.

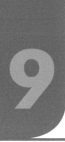

9 Laparoscopic Radical Cystoprostatectomy

POSITION

- The patient is positioned supine for draping and trocar insertion.
- The rest of the procedure is performed in Trendelenburg position with the legs straight and both arms are alongside the body (Figure 9.1).

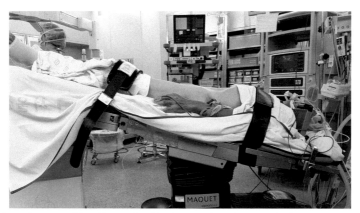

Figure 9.1 Trendelenburg position. The patient is strapped and supported; pressure areas are padded; electrocautery is connected; flatus tube is inserted; intermittent pneumatic calf compression device and elastic stocking are applied. Arms are wrapped and padded to the patient's side.

- Straps and adhesives are applied to support and stabilize the patient.
- Flatus tube is introduced into the rectum and a nasogastric tube is inserted if the intestine will be used for urinary diversion.
- A urethral catheter is inserted in the sterile draped field.

PORT INSERTION

- The ports are inserted in a straight supine position.
- Veress needle is introduced through a 1.5-cm midline abdominal incision, 4 cm above the umbilicus.

Confirmation of Veress needle passage and position is explained in Chapter 3, Section 1 "Basic Instrumentation".

DOI: 10.1201/b22928-11

- Pneumoperitoneum is created to 15 mmHg for trocar insertion after which it is set down to 12 mmHg throughout the procedure.
- An 11-mm trocar is inserted at the Veress needle site and a 10-mm laparoscope with 30° lens is introduced to assess:

  - Veress needle and port entry area for injuries
  - Presence of adhesions
  - Main landmarks and critical structures
  - Entry sites for next ports

Access can also be obtained using the open (Hasson) technique or by direct vision using an optiview trocar with the laparoscope.

- Another four trocars are inserted at about 15 cm from the symphysis pubis in a fan-shaped (hemicircular) configuration toward the pelvis, keeping around 7 cm in-between (Figure 9.2).

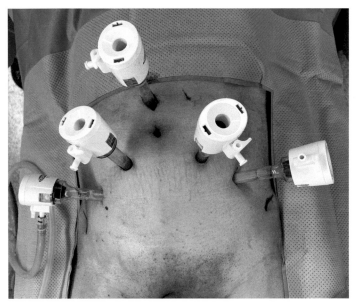

Figure 9.2 Port configurations.

- All ports are 11 mm except the right paramedian port where a 12-mm trocar is used for 12-mm Endo-GIA bladder pedicle stapling.

> In case of cutaneous ureterostomy or ileal conduit diversion is being planned, and the skin at the right paramedian port site is circumferentially (2 cm diameter) excised before trocar insertion.

OPERATING ROOM SETUP AND SURGEON POSITIONS

- The operating room is set up to facilitate a smooth flow of surgery (Figure 9.3).
- The surgeon operates from the left side of the patient.
- The first assistant stands at the right side of the patient, holding the camera and using the right side ports for assistance.
- A second assistant stands at the right side of the patient, using the far lateral port and taking care of catheter manipulation.

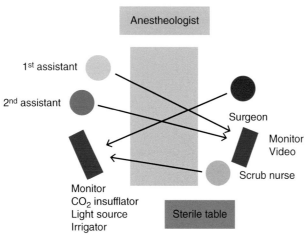

Figure 9.3 Diagram of the operation room setup showing the surgical team positions in relation to the patient, monitors and the accessory machines.

STEP-BY-STEP SURGERY

URETERIC DISSECTION

- At Trendelenburg position, the intestine is further retracted cranially and bowel adhesions at the pelvis and the dissection area are lysed if present (Figure 9.4).

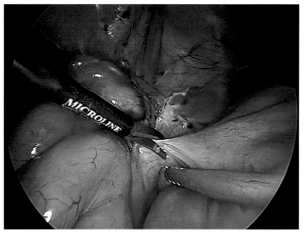

Figure 9.4 Adhesiolysis of bowel adhesions to the pelvic side wall (right).

- Starting from either side, the peritoneum over the common iliac artery bifurcation is opened using monopolar scissors.
- The leaflet of the peritoneum is grasped by the assistant through a right side port and retracted (Figure 9.5).
- The peritoneum incision is widened and the attachment to ureter is released using ultrasonic shear (Thunderbeat).
- The peritoneal incision is extended along the course of the ureter toward the bladder distally and medially to the rectovesical reflection (Figure 9.6).
- The ureter is dissected circumferentially and released from the surrounding attachment using an energy device, keeping the periureteric tissue and vasculature intact.

Take care to avoid direct grasping of the ureter or applying coagulation on its wall, which may compromise its vasculature.

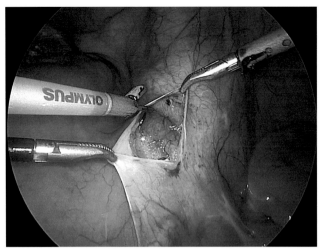

Figure 9.5 Opening the peritoneum on the bifurcation of common iliac artery (right). The peritoneal leaflets are grasped and retracted.

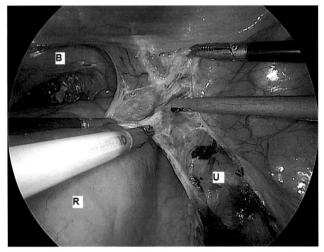

Figure 9.6 Peritoneal incision extension along the course of the ureter (U) to the bladder (B) (right side). *Abbreviation:* R, rectum.

- Proximally, the left ureter is extensively mobilized to the maximum level where the instruments can reach.

Long proximal left ureter-free length is necessary for providing a tension-free ureteral anastomosis during urinary diversion, after its transposition to the right side, crossing posterior to the sigmoid mesentery.

- The first assistant provides a wide exposure by retracting the sigmoid colon medially away from the dissection field.

To facilitate the dissection and to free the surgeon's left hand, the ureter is grasped by the second assistant with Babcock forceps and is manipulated to expose the dissection plane (Figure 9.7).

- The gonadal vessels can be identified crossing laterally anterior to the ureter toward the internal inguinal ring.
- They are isolated and clipped, if interfering with ureteric dissection.
- Distally, the ureter is dissected until the level of the ureteric hiatus on the bladder.

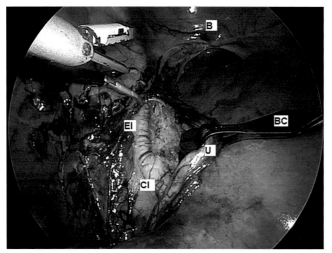

Figure 9.7 Gentle retraction of the ureter (U) by babcock forceps (BC). *Abbreviations*: B, bladder; CI, common iliac artery; EI, external iliac artery (left side).

Ureteric mobilization until the bladder will facilitate identification and control of the vascular pedicle at later steps.

- The vas deference crosses the ureter anteriorly near the bladder. It is clipped by M-size Hem-o-lok and divided (Figure 9.8).

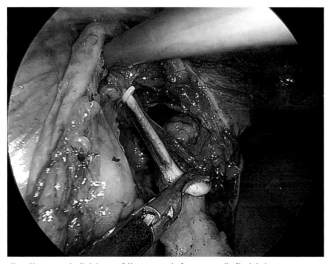

Figure 9.8 Isolation, ligation and division of the vas deference (left side).

Just distal to the crossing vas, a branch from superior vesical artery is usually identified anteriorly. It can be cauterized or clipped and divided (Figure 9.9).

The ureteric dissection usually comes to end once it crosses the vas and superior vesical artery.

- The ureter is clipped at most distal part by two XL-size Hem-o-lok clips and divided in-between (Figure 9.10).

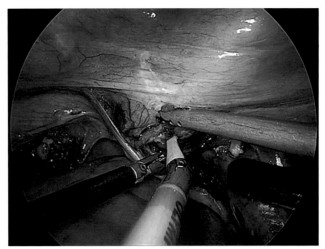

Figure 9.9 Arterial branch from superior vesical artery is transected by ultrasonic shear device.

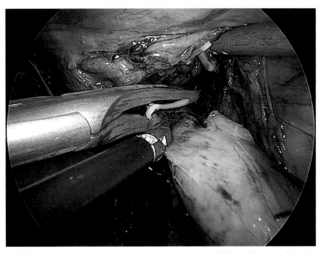

Figure 9.10 Clipping of the ureter. Note the angle orientation of the clip applicator.

Early clipping of the ureter allows for hydrodistension, which may facilitate easy anastomosis during diversion.

- A frozen section for histological examination is sent from the proximal ureteric stump and the ureter is placed in the upper abdomen to avoid injury during the rest of procedure.

The same is performed for the other side ureter.

POSTERIOR DISSECTION

- The peritoneum is incised horizontally at the rectovesical reflection connecting the previous peritoneal incisions of ureteric dissection.

Posterior dissection is performed before the anterior peritoneal and Retzius space dissection to prevent the fall of the bladder on the field.

- Dissection toward the seminal vesicles and the vasa deferentia is carried out in a loose areolar fatty tissue plane (Figure 9.11).

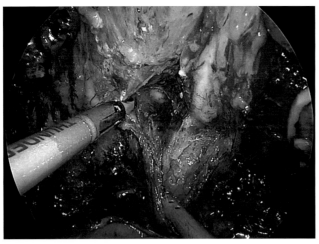

Figure 9.11 Posterior dissection.

Take care to avoid anterior dissection on the bladder or deep on the rectum posteriorly.

- The posterior peritoneal flab is retracted down by the assistant section device for maximum exposure.
- If difficulty is encountered finding the seminal vesicle, the previously transected vas deference is grasped anteriorly and dissected distally toward the prostate.
- The blood vessels and posterior connective tissue attachment of both the seminal vesicle and the vas are cauterized and peeled off (Figure 9.12).

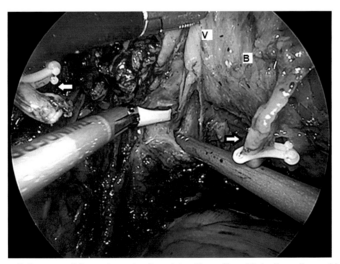

Figure 9.12 Left vas deference (V) and seminal vesicle dissection. Note the clipped left and right vasa (arrows). The rectum is seen posteriorly. *Abbreviation*: B, bladder.

- The vas and seminal vesicle are retracted anteriorly by the second assistant locking grasper, and the posterior dissection is continued until the base of the prostate.
- The Denonvilliers' fascia is seen stretched posteriorly; its attachment to prostate is opened horizontally and an intra-fascial plane is created if nerve sparing approach is planned (Figure 9.13).
- If nerve sparing is not planned, then the plane of dissection will be extra-fascial between the Denonvilliers' fascia and perirectal fat.

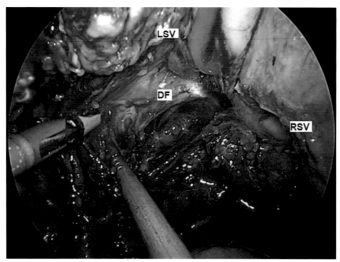

Figure 9.13 Denonvilliers' fascia (DF) dissection. Note the anterior traction of left seminal vesicle (LSV) and posterior down traction by suction probe. *Abbreviation*: RSV, right seminal vesicle.

DROPPING THE BLADDER AND RETZIUS SPACE DISSECTION

- The surgeon uses Maryland forceps through a left side port and monopolar scissors through the right paramedian port.
- The right medial umbilical ligament distal to the umbilicus level is retracted down by the left Maryland.
- The peritoneum is incised horizontally using monopolar scissors just lateral and parallel to the ligament (Figure 9.14).

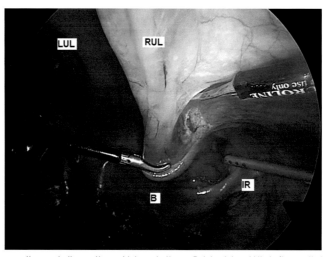

Figure 9.14 Anterior peritoneal dissection. *Abbreviations*: B, bladder; LUL, left medial umbilical ligament; IR, right internal inguinal ring; RUL, right medial umbilical ligament.

- A plane of loose areolar tissue will form between the peritoneum and transversalis fascia (Figure 9.15).

The dissection is carried out through the areolar tissue plane on the peritoneum and take care not to dissect superficially on the transversalis fascia.

- The assistant can further retract down the peritoneum by a suction device while clearing up the smoke.
- The same step is performed for the left medial umbilical ligament using the two left side ports (Secteroization).
- The two umbilical ligaments incisions are connected and the urachus is transected at the level of the umbilicus.

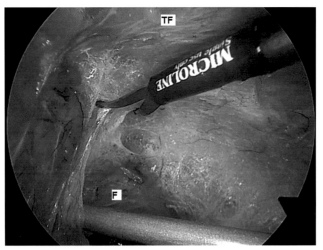

Figure 9.15 Anterior peritoneal dissection is performed through the areolar fatty plane avoiding the transversalis fascia (TF) anteriorly. *Abbreviation*: F, extraperitoneal fat.

- The peritoneum is incised as an inverted V shape following the medial umbilical ligaments until meeting the previously opened posterior peritoneum (Figure 9.16).

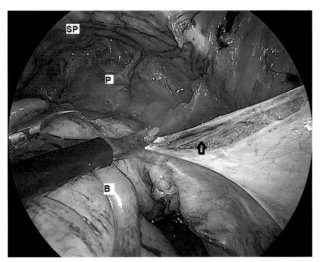

Figure 9.16 The anterior peritoneal incision along the vas deference (arrow) meeting the posterior incision. Note the Retzius space, B, bladder. *Abbreviations*: P, prostate; SP, symphysis pubis.

- The dissection in the plane of gray loose areolar tissue is continued until the bony pelvis, anterior to the bladder and prostate (Retzius space).

> Dissecting far lateral to the medial umbilical ligament and internal inguinal ring landmarks may injure the inferior epigastric vessels.

No need to clip the vas at this level as it has already been clipped and divided during distal ureteric dissection.

- The lateral bladder wall is dissected off the lateral pelvic wall fat through a relatively avascular plane by sweeping movement with blunt and sharp dissection (Figure 9.17).

Take care to avoid injury to the external iliac vessels and obturator nerve on lateral pelvic wall.

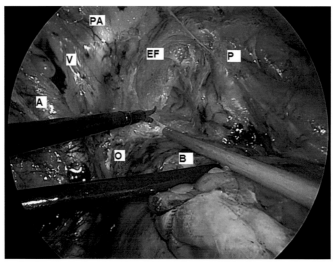

Figure 9.17 Lateral bladder wall mobilization. *Abbreviations*: A, external iliac artery; B, bladder; EF, endopelvic fascia; O, obturator nerve; P, prostate; PA, pelvic arch; V, external iliac vein (Left side).

DEFATTING THE PROSTATE AND ENDOPELVIC FASCIA

- The fat overlaying the endopelvic fascia and prostate is swept off and rolled medially toward the bladder neck (Figure 9.18).

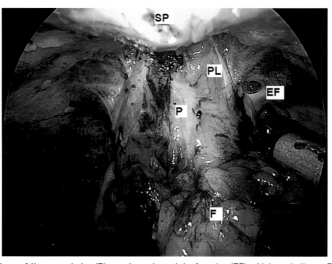

Figure 9.18 Defatting of the prostate (P) and endopelvic fascia (EF). *Abbreviations*: F, dissected fat; PL, puboprostatic ligament; SP, symphysis pubis.

- The superficial dorsal vein is identified in the fat between the two puboprostatic ligaments. It is isolated, cauterized and transected.

The purpose of defatting the prostate and endopelvic fascia:

1. Visualizing the puboprostatic ligament overlaying the dorsal vascular complex (DVC).
2. Defining the prostatic contour and its apex.
3. Accurate opening of endopelvic fascia lateral to prostate.

OPENING THE ENDOPELVIC FASCIA

- The endopelvic fascia is incised lateral to the prostate just distal to the bladder neck (Figure 9.19).

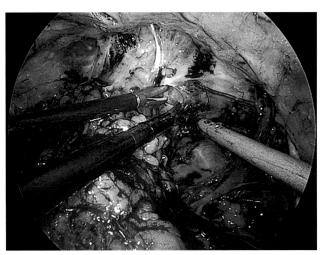

Figure 9.19 Opening the endopelvic fascia (right side).

- The levator muscle within the layers of endopelvic fascia is swept and peeled off the prostate toward the pelvic wall without cautery (Figure 9.20).

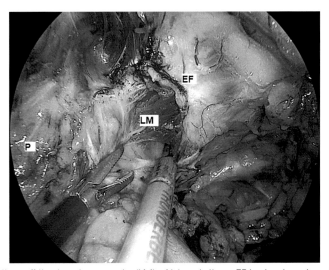

Figure 9.20 Dissecting off the levator muscle (LM). *Abbreviations*: EF, incised endopelvic fascia; P, prostate.

Take care to avoid the large dilated veins of the prostatic fascia on the lateral wall of the prostate, medial to endopelvic fascial incision.

- Endopelvic fascia incision is extended toward the prostatic apex where the puboprostatic ligament is transected and apical muscular attachment is identified and released.

> Puboprostatic ligament division is important to clearly visualize the apical muscular attachment, prostatic apex and DVC.

- The distal apical lateral muscle attachment may contain a small vessel. It is coagulated and transected on the prostatic surface by an energy device and swept off to the pelvic wall (Figure 9.21).

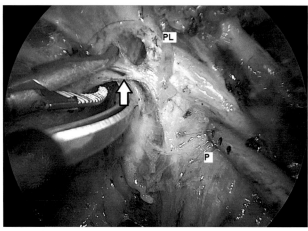

Figure 9.21 Transection of left puboprostatic ligament (PL). Note the apical attachment contains a blood vessel (arrow). *Abbreviation*: P, prostate.

The same steps are performed for the other side.

DORSAL VASCULAR COMPLEX LIGATION

- Once the puboprostatic ligament is incised and the apex is cleared from the muscular attachment, the DVC will be clearly seen.
- A 20-cm PDS stitch on 1/2 circle, 31-mm MH-1 needle is used for DVC ligation.
- The needle is horizontally oriented with its curve parallel to the pubic arch (Figure 9.22).

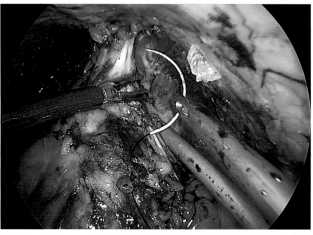

Figure 9.22 The needle orientation and introduction perpendicular to DVC. Note the retraction.

- The needle is introduced through the plane between DVC and the urethra from right to left using wrist rotation (pronation movement).

For optimum exposure during needle introduction, the surgeon's left hand retracts the prostatic apex to the left while the assistant retracts on the bladder neck level.

- Once the needle pierces the right side, the left side is exposed by the assistant suction device retracting on the apex to the right and the needle exit is adjusted (Figure 9.23).

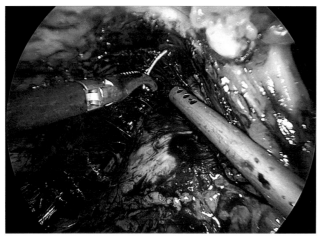

Figure 9.23 Needle exit from the left side of DVC. Note the retraction by suction probe.

- The needle is carefully removed by its curve to avoid DVC injury and bleeding.
- The DVC is ligated as a figure of 8 with a slipped knot to ensure a tight closure (Chapter 4, Figure 4.20).

THE BLADDER PEDICLE CONTROL

> After ureteric mobilization and anterolateral peritoneal dissection, the bladder will be only attached posterolaterally by the pedicle.

- To clearly visualize the pedicle, the bladder is retracted anteromedially to the contralateral side.
- The pedicle is seen as a punch of stretched tissue posterolaterally distal to the obliterated umbilical artery (medial umbilical ligament) (Figure 9.24).

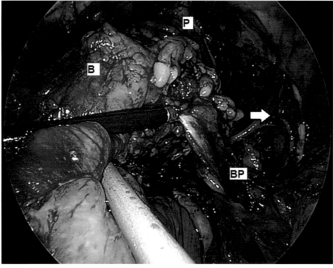

Figure 9.24 Isolation and preparation of the right bladder pedicle for ligation. Obutrator neurovascular bundle (arrow). *Abbreviations*: B, bladder; P, prostate. Note the bladder countertraction.

- The pedicle is controlled by using a 12-mm Endo-GIA Ultra stapler (Covidien) introduced through right pararectus 12-mm port.
- The GIA can be adjusted by rotating and angulating the articulating jaws to include maximum length of the pedicle with the obliterated umbilical artery (Figure 9.25).

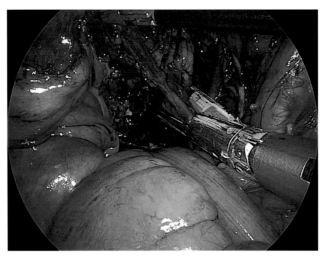

Figure 9.25 Control of the left bladder pedicle using GIA vascular stapler.

To prevent GIA malfunctioning or misfiring resulting in bleeding, it is important to exclude any interfering clips in-between the jaws.

- The obliterated umbilical artery (medial umbilical ligament) can be clipped and divided separately.
- Sequential GIA control and transection may be required in long pedicles.
- The residual attachment of the pedicle at the distal stapled line is clipped by an L-size Hem-o-lok and divided by scissors.

Dividing the stapled tissue attachment using ultrasonic shears will spoil the device due the metallic staples.

> The pedicle can alternatively be controlled by multiple Hem-o-lok clips and divided by an energy device.

- The same steps are followed for the other side of the bladder pedicle.

THE PROSTATE PEDICLE AND NERVE SPARING

- The dissection is directed to the prostatic pedicle which may not be included in the GIA staple line.

As the bladder falls down after anterior dissection, approaching the prostatic pedicle posteriorly may be difficult and challenging.

- With contralateral traction of the bladder and prostate, the prostatic pedicle can be seen identified stretched posterolaterally at the end of the stapled line of the bladder pedicle.
- The pedicel is controlled by L-size Hem-o-loks and divided by cold scissors toward the prostate (Figure 9.26).
- The seminal vesicle is retracted anteromedially by the assistant locking grasper and the plane above Denonvilliers' fascia which was created posteriorly is identified.

> The neurovascular bundle (NVB) lies between prostatic fascia and levator fascia, so the nerve sparing approach is carried out in the intrafacial plane (between the prostatic capsule and prostatic fascia).

- The posterior plane between the prostate and Denonvilliers' fascia is connected by a right angle to the lateral plane (between the prostatic capsule and prostatic fascia) (Figure 9.27).

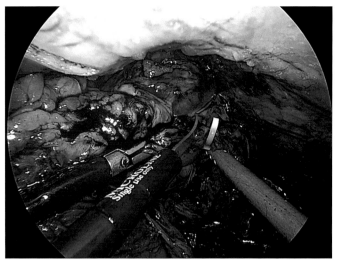

Figure 9.26 Right prostatic pedicle ligation by Hem-o-lok clip and division by cold scissors.

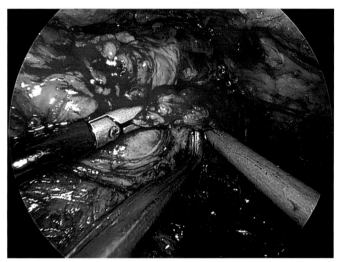

Figure 9.27 Intrafascial plane is created between the prostatic capsule and prostatic fascia using a right-angled dissector (right side).

- From the posterolateral edge (horn) of the prostate, the levator and prostatic fascia are peeled off from the prostatic capsule using cold scissors as in nerve sparing radical prostatectomy.
- The dissection is continued in anterolateral direction until the prostatic apex (Figure 9.28).

Electrocautery should be avoided if nerve sparing is intended.

- If nerve sparing is not planned, then the dissection sill be extra-fascial.
- Bleeding from the dilated periprostatic veins may occur. It usually stops spontaneously, avoiding unnecessary electrocautery.

The same is performed for the other side of the prostate.

DIVISION OF DVC AND URETHRA

- The DVC is divided on the prostatic apex using monopolar scissors or energy device until the urethra.
- The periurethral tissue and muscular attachment are cleared from the urethra circumferentially by using blunt and sharp dissection.
- Once the urethra is freed anterolaterally, a posterior window is created by a right-angled dissector.

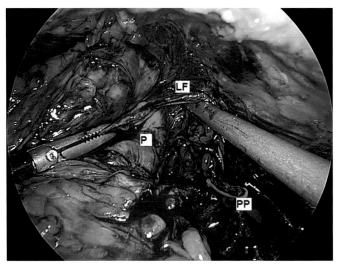

Figure 9.28 Nerve sparing. Peeling the prostatic and levator fascia (LF) from the prostate (P). Countertraction by assistant suction probe facilitates the dissection. *Abbreviation*: PP, clipped prostatic pedicle (right).

- A vessel loop is placed around the urethra and retracted upward and cranially to clearly visualize its sides (Figure 9.29).

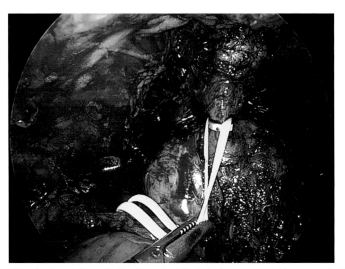

Figure 9.29 The urethra is circumferentially dissected, isolated on a vessel loop and clipped proximally on the prostate.

- The Foley catheter is removed and the urethra is clipped (*to prevent tumor cell spillage*) toward the prostate by an XL-size Hem-o-lok and divided by cold scissors close to the clip.
- The distal urethra can be clamped if orthotopic bladder is not planned.
- A frozen section is sent from the proximal urethral stump distal to the clip.
- Rectaurethralis and residual Denonvilliers' fascia attachment to the prostatic apex are released gently and carefully (Figure 9.30).

Rectal tenting during removal of the prostate due to posterior apical attachment keeps the rectum at risk of injury.

- The specimen is placed in an XL-size endo-catch bag and the thread is clipped to ensure closure.

Pelvic lymph nodes dissection is performed after this step (Figure 9.31).

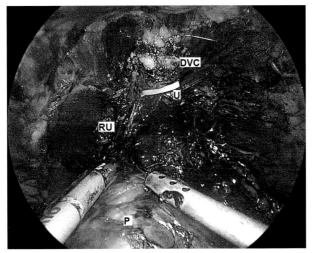

Figure 9.30 Releasing the residual rectourethralis (RU) attachment. *Abbreviations:* DVC, ligated deep vascular complex; P, prostate; U, clipped urethra.

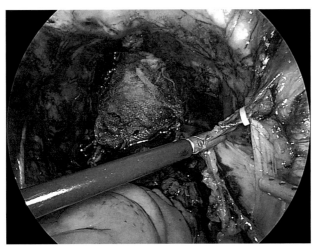

Figure 9.31 Left external iliac LN dissection.

TRANSPOSITION OF LEFT URETER TO THE RIGHT SIDE

- The left side of the sigmoid mesentery is dissected posteriorly and just anterior to the common iliac vessels (Figure 9.32).
- The sigmoid colon is retracted to the right side by the assistant retractors providing a maximum exposure.
- An adequate window is created posterior to the mesentery and the left ureter is transported through to the right side for urinary diversion.

Orthotopic urinary diversion is explained in Section 2, Chapter 10.

HEMOSTASIS, WOUND CLOSURE, DRAIN AND SPECIMEN REMOVAL

- The resection bed and lymph node (LN) dissection areas are reassessed for hemostasis.
- Active bleeding at the vascular pedicle or NVB can be secured by clips or by selective coagulation.
- The dissection area above the rectum is cleaned by suction irrigation and a hemostatic agent like FloSeal is applied.
- A drain is inserted and the port wounds (>10 mm) are closed using a Carter Thomason device.
- The specimen is removed through an extended camera port wound.

A detailed explanation of drain and closure along with figures is provided in Section 1.

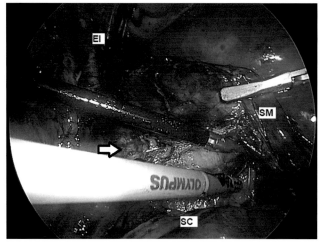

Figure 9.32 Transposition of the left ureter posterior to the sigmoid mesentery (SM) and anterior to common iliac artery (arrow). Note the mesentery retraction. *Abbreviations*: EI, external iliac artery; SC, sigmoid colon.

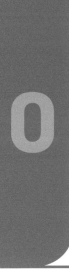

Extracorporeal Urinary Diversion (Modified Studer Orthotopic Ileal Neobladder) and Intracorporeal Urethra-Neobladder Anastomosis

STEP-BY-STEP SURGERY

ISOLATION OF AN ILEAL SEGMENT

- At the end of cystectomy, a stay stitch is taken on the ileum, around 15–20 cm proximal to the ileocecal junction.
- Another stay stitch is taken at the ureters, and both stay stitches are brought out of the abdomen.
- The midline supra-umbilical camera port wound is extended inferiorly below the umbilicus and the cystectomy specimen is extracted.
- The ileum and the ureters are brought out through the wound.
- Around 50 cm ileal segment proximal to the stay stitch is marked ensuring a free mobility of the segment to reach the symphysis pubis.

The measurement is taken at the mesoileal border to avoid incorrect length due to intestinal contraction.

- The mesentery is transilluminated by the operating table lighthead and the vascular arcades are visualized (Figure 10.1).
- The arterial arcades supplying the segment are identified and mesenteric windows between the branches are created toward the marked ileum.
- The branching vessels crossing the mesenteric windows are isolated on mosquito clamps, divided and ligated by 4/0 silk.

The arterial arcade selection and division for the neobladder segment should not jeopardize the blood supply of the ileum.

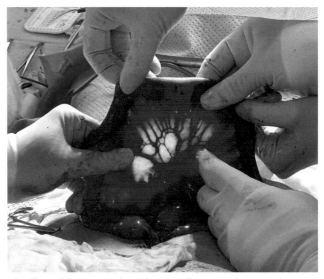

Figure 10.1 Transillumination of the mesentery showing the vascular arcades.

- The proximal and distal marked sites on the ileum in-between the divided mesentery are transected using 60–3.8-mm GIA stapler, DST series (Covidien) (Figure 10.2).

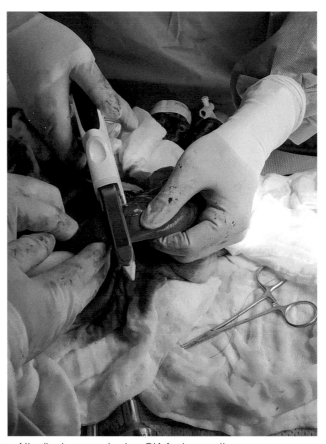

Figure 10.2 Isolation of the ileal segment using GIA for transection.

The area around the bowel is padded by large towels to prevent intraperitoneal contamination by intestinal contents.

RESTORATION OF THE INTESTINAL CONTINUITY

- The stapling lines of the proximal and distal ileum are transected and cleaned by betadine and saline cotton gauze.
- The continuity of the ileum is restored anterior to the isolated segment by side-to-side anastomosis at the antimesenteric borders using a GIA stapler (Figure 10.3).

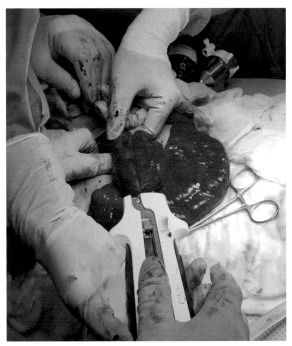

Figure 10.3 Side-to-side ileal anastomosis anterior to the isolated ileal segment using GIA.

For accurate anastomosis, it is essential to ensure correct wall alignment without a twist, avoiding any intervening mesenteric fat in-between the stapling lines.

- The anastomotic opened end is closed by GIA avoiding the overlap of staple lines (Figure 10.4).
- The ileal mesenteric window is closed and the ileum is introduced into the abdomen.

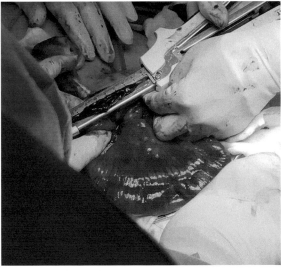

Figure 10.4 Closure of the ileal anastomosis.

- The stapled distal end of the isolated ileal segment is opened and irrigated by copious amount of normal saline until the drain is crystal clear (Figure 10.5).

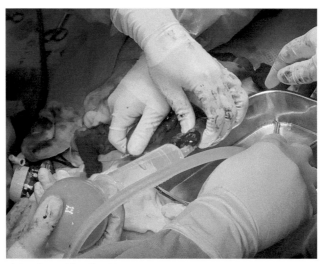

Figure 10.5 Copious irrigation of the ileal loop.

- The drained fluid is sucked out immediately from a kidney dish and the area is kept clean and dry.
- After completion of irrigation, all instruments used, towels and gloves are changed to avoid any possible contamination.
- Around 40 cm of the distal ileal loop is opened at the antimesenteric border leaving around 10 cm of the loop proximally intact as an afferent limb (Figure 10.6).

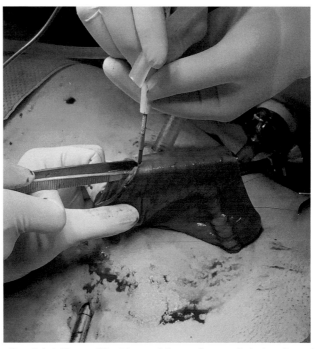

Figure 10.6 Opening the distal 40 cm of ileal loop at the antimesenteric border using cutting elctrocautery.

- The opened loop is configured in a U shape (Figure 10.7).

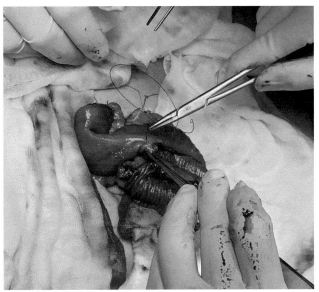

Figure 10.7 U-configuration of the opened loop. Note the proximal afferent closed loop.

- The medial (posterior) borders of the U is oversewn by continuous running suturing in two layers using a 3/0 V-Loc stitch (Figure 10.8).

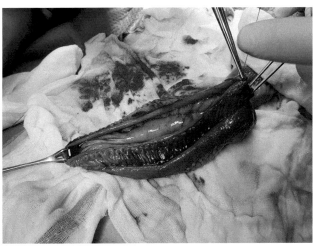

Figure 10.8 Medial (posterior) borders of the U are oversewn using the V-Loc stitch.

URETERO-ILEAL ANASTOMOSIS

- A 1.5-cm posterior spatulation is performed on both ureters.
- Two enterotomies for ureteral anastomosis are made by excising around 1.5 cm of intestinal wall at both sides of the afferent loop.
- Ureteroileal interrupted suturing anastomoses is performed using 5/0 Monosyn stitch on 1/2 circle, 13-mm HR needle.
- Ureteric catheters are inserted into the ureters to the kidney, brought out through the lateral walls of the loop and fixed by a stitch on the seromuscular layer.
- The ileal reservoir is closed by suturing the lateral (anterior) borders of the U loop anteriorly in two layers using 3/0 vicryl stitch (Figure 10.9).
- Around 2-cm diameter of neobladder neck is formed at the most distal end of the suture line (Figure 10.10).
- Keeping a long stay stitch at the bladder neck will facilitate intracorporeal manipulation, and the reservoir is introduced into the abdomen.

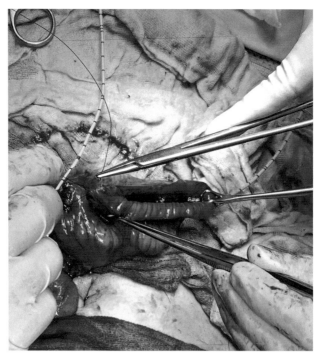

Figure 10.9 Closure of the reservoir by suturing the lateral (anterior) borders of the U loop.

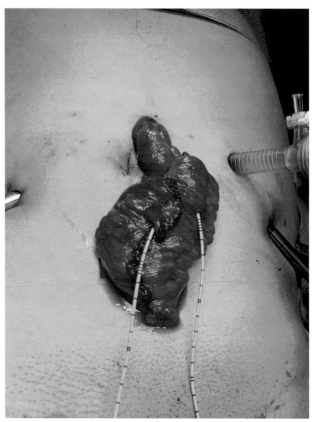

Figure 10.10 Neobladder neck is formed at the distal end of anterior suture line of the reservoir. The ureteric catheters are fixed to the ileal wall by vicryl stitch.

- The ureteric stents are brought out to the abdominal wall distal to midway between the left anterior-superior iliac spine and umbilicus and are fixed to the skin.
- The umbilical-wound fascia is partially closed using 1/0 vicryl, leaving a gap for the camera port.
- Alternatively a wound retractor device is fixed into the umbilical wound and pneumoperitoneum is created.
- The cystectomy dissection area at the pelvis is reassessed for hemostasis.

URETHRA-NEOBLADDER ANASTOMOSIS

- The reservoir is pulled down to the pelvic by the stay stitch on the neobladder neck (Figure 10.11).

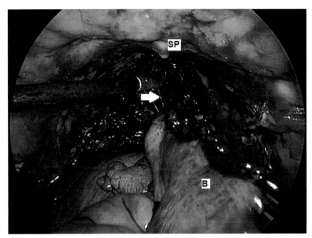

Figure 10.11 Introducing the neobladder reservoir (B) into the pelvis by pulling the bladder neck stay stitch (arrow). *Abbreviation*: SP, symphysis pubis.

- Urethra-neobladder anastomosis is performed using a 15-cm, 3/0 V-Loc stitch on a 17-mm 1/2 circle, CV-23 needle.
- Anastomosis starts at 5 o'clock position until 11 o'clock at the left side in a continuous running suturing (Figure 10.12).

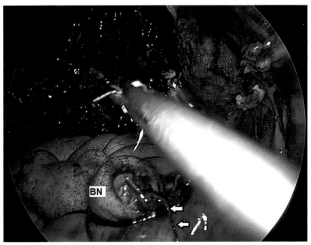

Figure 10.12 Urethra-neobladder anastomosis starting at 5 o'clock on the neobladder neck (BN). Stay stitch (arrows).

For every urethral stitch, the second assistant should manipulate the catheter tip in/out to open the urethra and guide the surgeon's needle (Figure 10.13).

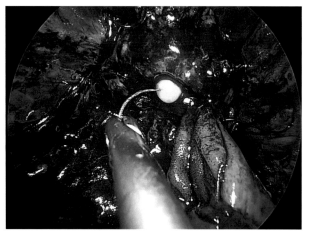

Figure 10.13 The needle is guided by the Foley catheter.

- After taking the bladder neck 6 o'clock stitch, the suture line is tightened, approximating the neobladder to the urethra.

Throughout the anastomosis, the suturing is always outside-in at the bladder and inside-out at the urethra.

For precise left side suturing from 7 to 11 o'clock:

- The bladder outside-in is performed by the left hand.
- The urethral inside-out is performed by the right hand (Figure 10.14).

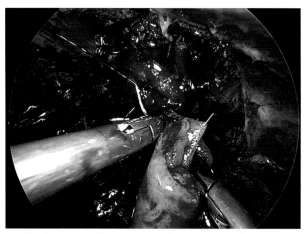

Figure 10.14 Left side (7–11 o'clock) urethra-neobladder anastomosis. Outside-in at the neobladder neck by left hand.

- Once left side anastomosis reaches 11 o'clock, another V-Loc stitch is introduced to start suturing the right side from 4 o'clock to 12 o'clock.

For right side precise suturing from 4 to 12 o'clock:

- The bladder outside-in is performed by the right hand.
- The urethral inside-out is performed by the left hand (Figure 10.15).

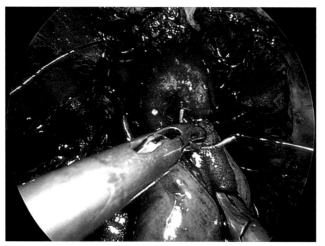

Figure 10.15 Right side (4–12 o'clock) urethra-neobladder anastomosis. Inside-out at the urethra by left hand.

To avoid tearing of the urethral wall while pulling out the thread, it should be pulled straight perpendicular to the wall which can be further supported by the other hand instrument (Figure 10.16).

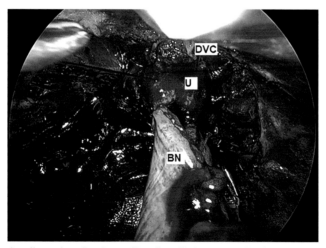

Figure 10.16 Tightening the suture line by pulling the stitch perpendicular to the urethral wall. *Abbreviations*: BN, neobladder neck; DVC, ligated deep vascular complex; U, urethra.

- The residual anterior bladder neck gap can be closed by the remaining right side anastomosis stitch before tying it with the left one.

During this step, the second assistant should make sure that the urethral catheter is not entrapped by the stitch and is moving freely in and out.

- The anastomosis integrity for leakage is assessed by filling the bladder to 100 mL of normal saline.
- For the purpose of achieving early continence recovery, an anterior sling from the bladder neck to symphysis pubis anteriorly is performed using the same stitch.

Robot-Assisted Urologic Surgery

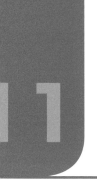

Transperitoneal Robot-Assisted Laparoscopic Radical Prostatectomy

POSITION

- The patient is positioned supine for draping and trocar insertion.
- The rest of the procedure is performed in Trendelenburg position with the legs straight and both arms are well wrapped and padded alongside the body.
- Straps and adhesives are applied to support and stabilize the patient (Figure 11.1).
- Flatus tube is introduced into the rectum and a urethral catheter is inserted in the sterile draped field.

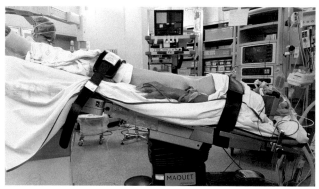

Figure 11.1 Trendelenburg position: the patient is strapped and supported; pressure areas are padded; electrocautery is connected; flatus tube is inserted; intermittent pneumatic calf compression device and elastic stocking are applied. Arms are wrapped and padded to the patient's side.

PORT INSERTION

- The trocars are inserted in a straight supine position.
- Veress needle is introduced through a 12-mm midline abdominal incision, 2 cm above the umbilicus.

Confirmation of Veress needle passage and correct position is explained in Chapter 3, Section 1 "Basic Instrumentation".

- Pneumoperitoneum is created to 15 mmHg for trocar insertion after which it is set to 12 mmHg throughout the procedure.

Access can also be obtained using the open (Hasson) technique or by direct vision using an optiview trocar with the laparoscope.

DOI: 10.1201/b22928-14

- A robotic 8-mm camera port is inserted at the Veress needle site.
- A da Vinci Xi 0° lens laparoscope is introduced to assess:

  - Veress needle and port entry area for injuries
  - Presence of adhesions
  - Main landmarks and critical structures
  - Entry sites of the next ports

- Another five port sites are marked using a ruler and the trocars are inserted (Figure 11.2).

  - Three Da Vinci Xi 8-mm robotic ports
  - Two assistant 11-mm disposable ports in the left side

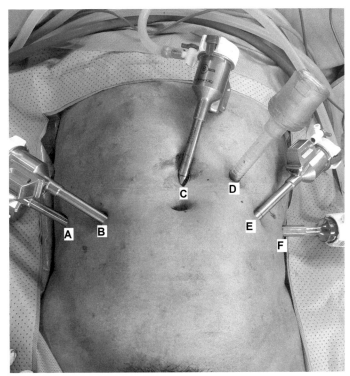

Figure 11.2 The trocar configurations. *Abbreviations*: A, arm 4 ProGrasp; B, arm 3 right-hand monopolar curved scissors; C, arm 2 camera; D, assistant right hand; E, arm 1 left-hand grasper; F, assistant left hand.

For the far lateral port, to avoid bowel injury, the intestine can be retracted during trocar insertion using a fan retractor.

DOCKING THE ROBOT AND INSERTING THE INSTRUMENTS

- After trocar insertions, the patient is positioned in a steep Trendelenburg position.
- The robotic cart is allocated to the right side of the patient and the camera is docked for targeting and repositioning before docking the other ports.

THE FOUR ROBOTIC ARMS

#1   Maryland Bipolar Forceps, Fenestrated (left hand)
#2   Camera: 0°
#3   Hot shear monopolar curved scissors (right hand)
#4   ProGrasp forceps

OPERATING ROOM SETUP AND ASSISTANT SURGEON POSITIONS

- The operating room is set up to facilitate a smooth flow of surgery (Figure 11.3).
- The first assistant:

  - *Position*: At the left side of the patient, using two 11-mm ports.
  - *Role*: Retraction, suction of blood and gas, changing robotic arms, cleaning the lens, applying clips, introducing and taking out instruments and supplies.

- A second assistant, when necessary:

  - *Position*: At the right side of the patient.
  - *Role*: Catheter care and manipulation, bladder filling and changing instruments.

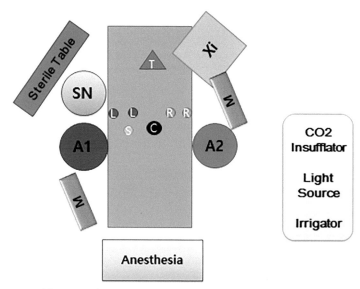

Figure 11.3 Diagram of the operation room setup showing the surgical team positions in relation to the patient, monitors (M), robotic cart (Xi) and accessory machines. *Abbreviations*: A, assistants; C, camera; R, L, right and left ports; S, suction; SN, scrub nurse; T, target organ.

STEP-BY-STEP SURGERY

ADHESIOLYSIS

- The intestine is retracted cranially from the pelvis and bowel adhesions at the pelvic side wall or at the dissection area are lysed if present (Figure 11.4).

> In addition to the Trendelenburg position, releasing the adhesions will further empty the pelvis for safe dissection. It will also prevent bowel injuries by the assistant instruments coming through the left side ports to the pelvis.

DROPPING THE BLADDER AND ENTERING THE RETZIUS SPACE

- The right medial umbilical ligament is retracted down just distal to the umbilicus using the fourth arm ProGrasp.
- The peritoneum is incised horizontally using hot shear scissor just lateral and parallel to the ligament (Figure 11.5).
- The dissection is carried out at the areolar tissue plane between the peritoneum and transversalis fascia (Figure 11.6).

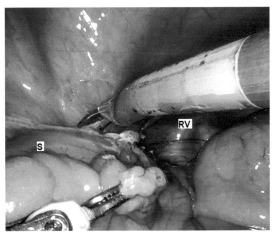

Figure 11.4 Adhesiolysis of the sigmoid colon at the pelvic left side wall. *Abbreviations*: RV, rectovesical pouch; S, sigmoid colon.

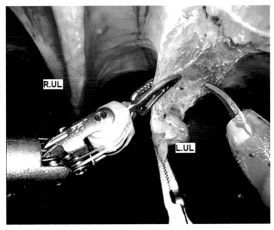

Figure 11.5 Anterior peritoneum is incised just lateral and parallel to right medial umbilical ligament (R.UL). *Abbreviation*: L.UL, left medial umbilical ligament.

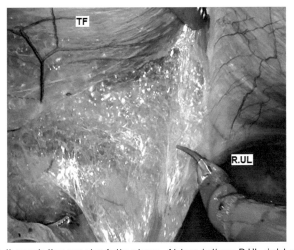

Figure 11.6 Dissection through the areolar fatty plane. *Abbreviations*: R.UL, right medial umbilical ligament; TF, transversalis fascia.

Care to avoid superficial dissection on the transversalis fascia anteriorly.

- The ProGrasp is repositioned to retract down both ligaments to transect the urachus and the left umbilical ligament is incised laterally.
- The assistant can further retract down the peritoneal flap by suction device while clearing up the smoke.

In addition to the Trendelenburg position, releasing the adhesions will further empty the pelvis for safe dissection. It will also prevent bowel injuries by the assistant instruments coming through the left side ports to the pelvis.

- The peritoneum is incised as an inverted V shape following the medial umbilical ligaments until crossing the vas deference medial to the internal inguinal ring (Figure 11.7).

Dissecting lateral to the medial umbilical ligament and internal inguinal ring landmarks may injure the inferior epigastric vessels.

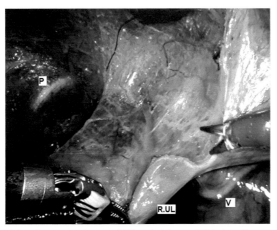

Figure 11.7 Peritoneal incision from urachus until the right vas (V) laterally, medial to the internal inguinal ring. *Abbreviations*: P, pubic ramus; R.UL, right umbilical ligament.

- The vas is isolated, clipped by M-size Hem-o-lok and transected by hot shear monopolar scissors (Figure 11.8).

Dissecting lateral to the medial umbilical ligament and internal inguinal ring landmarks may injure the inferior epigastric vessels.

- The dissection in the plane of gray loose areolar tissue is continued until the bony pelvis, anterior to the bladder and prostate.
- From the level of clipped vas, the lateral bladder wall is dissected off the lateral pelvic wall fat through a relatively avascular plane by sweeping movement with blunt and sharp dissection (Figure 11.9).

Releasing the lateral bladder wall from the pelvic side wall will provide an extra bladder mobility and facilitate a tension-free vesicourethral anastomosis.

Take care to avoid injury to the ureter, external iliac vessels and obturator nerve on lateral pelvic wall (Figure 11.10).

Step-by-Step Surgery

153

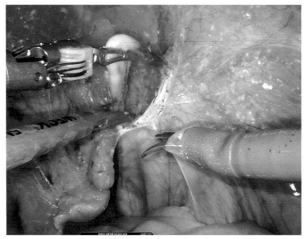

Figure 11.8 Isolation, clip ligation and division of the right vas deference.

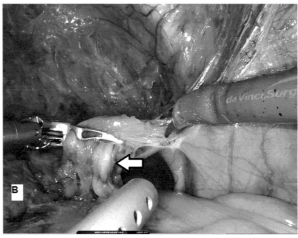

Figure 11.9 Dissecting the lateral bladder attachment from the pelvic walls. Clipped right vas deference (arrow). *Abbreviation:* B, bladder.

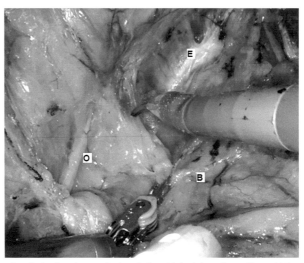

Figure 11.10 Attention to vitals structures during lateral bladder dissection. *Abbreviations:* B, bladder; E, endopelvic fasica; O, obturator nerve (left side).

DEFATTING THE PROSTATE AND ENDOPELVIC FASCIA

- The areolar tissue attaching the prostate to the pelvic wall is cleared by blunt and sharp dissection (Figure 11.11).
- The fourth arm ProGrasp retracts the bladder and prostate to the opposite side.

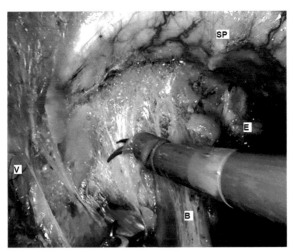

Figure 11.11 Dissecting the fatty attachment on left endopelvic fascia. Note the cleared right endopelvic fascia (E). *Abbreviations*: B, bladder; SP, symphysis pubis; V, left external iliac vein.

Take care not to injure the accessory pudendal artery which, if present, may be identified laterally above the endopelvic fascia (Figure 11.12).

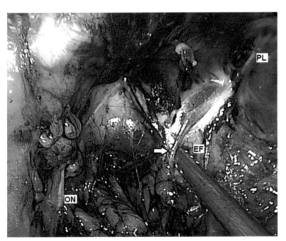

Figure 11.12 Accessory pudendal artery (arrow) on the endopelvic fascia (EF). *Abbreviations*: ON, left obturator nerve; PL, left puboprostatic ligament.

- The fat overlaying the endopelvic fascia and prostate is swept off and rolled medially and proximally toward the bladder.
- While defatting the prostatic apex, the superficial dorsal vein is identified between the two puboprostatic ligaments. It is isolated, cauterized and transected (Figure 11.13).

> The prostatic fat is light and easily removed compared to adherent fat of the bladder; demarcating the vesicoprostatic junction.

- The fat is excised and kept at the left iliac fossa to be included later with the specimen.

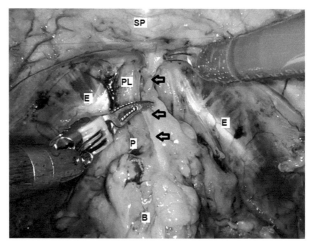

Figure 11.13 Defatting of the prostate and cauterization of superficial dorsal vein (arrows). *Abbreviations*: B, bladder; E, defatted endopelvic fascia; P, prostate; PL, puboprostatic ligament; SP, symphysis pubis.

Venous bleeding encountered while removing the prostatic fat at level of bladder neck is usually of the superficial dorsal vein extension.

The purpose of removing prostatic and endopelvic fat:

* Demarcating vesicoprostatic junction.
* Visualizing the puboprostatic ligament overlying the dorsal vascular complex (DVC).
* Defining the prostatic contour.
* Facilitating the dissection of bladder neck.
* For histopathology examination.

Accurate Opening of Endopelvic Fascia (If DVC Ligation Is Planned).

DORSAL VASCULAR COMPLEX (DVC)

* In robotic prostatectomy, the DVC is not ligated until prostatectomy is done; so the puboprostatic ligament is not divided and the endopelvic fascia is spared.

Detailed endopelvic fascia incision and DVC ligation is discussed in Chapter 4.

BLADDER NECK DISSECTION

The ways for defining the bladder neck:

1. Margin between loose fat of prostate and adherent fat of bladder.
2. Consistency difference between prostate and bladder.
3. Bladder neck outlined by the catheter balloon under traction.
4. The crossing fibers of puboprostatic ligaments meet at vesicoprostatic junction (varies between patients).

---

* Bladder detrusor apron over the base of the prostate is grasped by the Maryland and the bladder neck is transected at this level using monopolar scissors (Figure 11.14).
* Gentle down traction on the bladder by the fourth arm will facilitate the bladder neck transection and visualize the muscle fibers.

Preserving the bladder neck is not mandatory, and transecting it proximally is less hazardous than having a positive margin. Furthermore, wider bladder neck will facilitate the vesicourethral anastomosis in the pelvis.

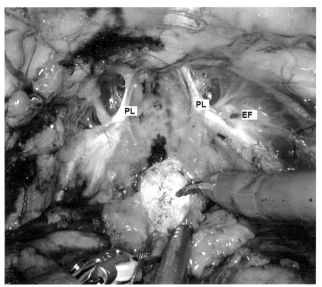

Figure 11.14 Transection of bladder neck by monopolar shears. *Abbreviations*: EF, right endopelvic fascia; PL, puboprostatic ligaments. Note the down traction by suction probe.

In large prostate or large median lobe, the configuration of the bladder neck may differ and incision site is changed accordingly.

Reviewing of preoperative MRI images is important to estimate the prostatic size and rule out asymmetric configuration.

- Once anterior bladder neck is transected, the urethral catheter tip is retracted anteriorly by the Pro-Grasp and the external part of the catheter is fixed to the drape.

This outward and upward traction of prostate by the urethral catheter will define the prostatic contour and facilitate the dissection.

- The posterior bladder neck mucosa is horizontally incised by hot shear scissors and the dissection is carried out on the margins of prostatic gland (Figure 11.15).

The lateral walls of bladder neck with perivesical fat are thinned out and flattened to easily facilitate the posterior mucosal incision and further deep dissection.

- The assistant should apply a gentle pressure on the anterior bladder neck to expose the posterior bladder neck wall and visualize the prostatic borders.
- If median lobe is encountered, the overlying mucosa is incised and the plane between the lobe and bladder wall is identified and dissected following the prostatic contour.
- This is facilitated by anterior traction of the median lobe using the fourth arm ProGrasp with the assistant countertracting the bladder neck posteriorly.

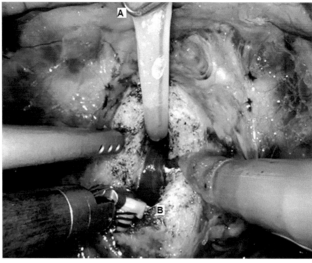

Figure 11.15 Transverse incision of posterior bladder neck mucosa by monopolar shears. A: Foley catheter retracted by ProGrasp; B: down traction of the bladder neck.

- The dissection is continued posteriorly until the longitudinal muscle fibers of bladder neck are transected (Figure 11.16).

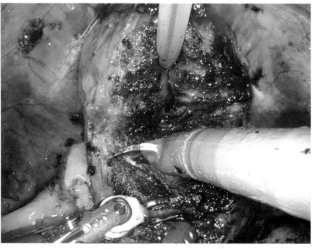

Figure 11.16 Transection of posterior longitudinal muscle fibers. The prostate is retracted by catheter and Maryland is retracting the posterior wall of bladder neck.

VAS DEFERENCE, SEMINAL VESICLES AND PROSTATIC PEDICLE

- The vasa and seminal vesicles are identified posterior to the thin longitudinal muscle fiber layers.

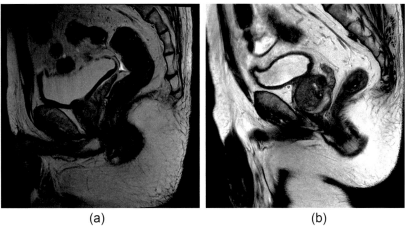

(a)   (b)

Figure 11.17 Sagittal sections of T2 MRI, showing the relationship between the bladder neck and seminal vesicle estimating the depth of dissection: (a) shallow and (b) deep.

- The vas deference (one side) is grasped out by the fourth arm and retracted anteriorly.
- The blood vessels and connective tissue attachment of the vas are cauterized and peeled off (Figure 11.18).
- The assistant's posterior countertraction by the suction device opens the space and ease the dissection.

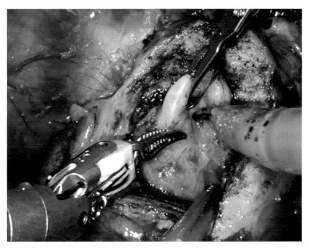

Figure 11.18 Dissection of left vas deference fibrovascular attachment by monopolar scissors. The vas is retracted anteriorly by ProGrasp with down traction by assistant suction device.

- The vas is transected by hot shear scissors and the distal stump is retracted to improve the seminal vesicle exposure.
- The seminal vesicle just lateral to the vas is gasped anteriorly by Maryland and dissected; sweeping off and cauterizing the blood vessels and connective tissue attachment (Figure 11.19).

To avoid any collateral thermal injuries to the posterolateral neurovascular bundle, the electrocautery if needed, is minimized and applied directly on the surface wall of the vas deference and seminal vesicles.

> Applying clips to the small vessels of the seminal vesicles and vas deference is not required. This is to avoid presence of foreign bodies near the urethrovesical anastomosis.

- The seminal vesicle is dissected until its junction with the prostate and with further anterior traction; the Denonvilliers' fascia will be clearly seen stretched posteriorly (Figure 11.20).

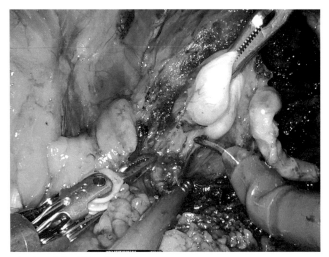

Figure 11.19 Left seminal vesicle (SV) dissection.

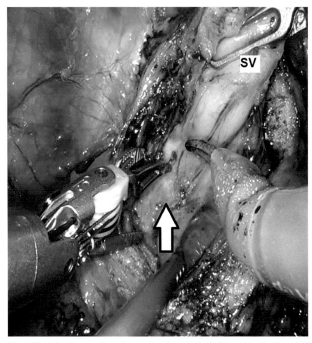

Figure 11.20 Denonvilliers' fascia (arrow), left seminal vesicle SV is retracted anteriorly by ProGrasp.

- Denonvilliers' fascia attachment is opened horizontally just posterior to the junction between seminal vesicle and prostate, aiming for intra-facial plane (if nerve sparing was planned).
- The intrafascial plane is created between the Denonvilliers' fascia and prostate (Figure 11.21).
- The dissection can be continued posterior to the prostate distally.
- The Denonvilliers' and prostatic fascia are released from the prostatic capsule by meticulous blunt and sharp dissection.
- To prevent capsular injury because of excessive traction, the small perforating vessels or fibrous attachment to the prostate are cauterized and/or divided.
- The assistant should provide a posterior downward countertraction on Denonvilliers' fascia.
- The prostatic pedicle which is seen stretched at the posterolateral edge of the prostate is dissected, thinned and clipped toward the prostate using L-size Hem-o-lok.

Take care to avoid deep posterior dissection or excessive downward pressure, which may perforate the fascia into the rectum.

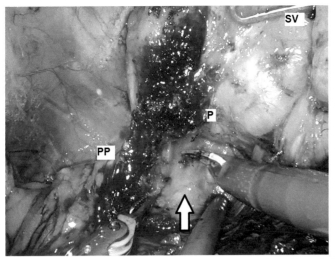

Figure 11.21 Intrafascial plane between the Denonvilliers' fascia (arrow) and prostatic capsule (P). Left prostatic pedicle PP. *Abbreviation*: SV, left seminal vesicle

NERVE SPARING

- Once the pedicle is clipped, it is divided by cold scissor close to the prostate and electrocautery is avoided.

The neurovascular bundle lies between prostatic fascia and levator fascia layers, and for nerve sparing, the dissection is performed at the intra-facial plane (between the prostatic capsule and prostatic fascia).

- The posterior intrafascial plane which has been already created above the Denonvilliers' fascia is connected by the scissors dissection to the lateral plane.
- From the posterolateral edge (horn) of the prostate, at the level of divided prostatic pedicle, the levator and prostatic fascia are peeled off from the prostatic capsule using cold scissors (Figure 11.22).

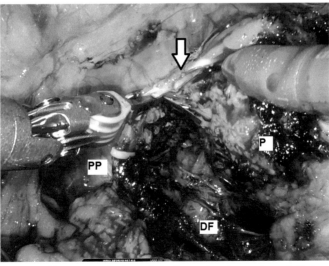

Figure 11.22 Nerve sparing. Neurovascular bundle between levator and prostatic fascia (arrow) is peeled off the prostatic capsule (P). Note the clipped pedicle (PP). *Abbreviation*: DF, Denonvilliers' fascia.

- Blunt and sharp dissection is continued in anterolateral direction until the puboprostatic ligament on the prostatic apex (Figure 11.23).
- The dissection is facilitated by contralateral counter traction of the prostate by the fourth arm Pro-Grasp on the seminal vesicle.

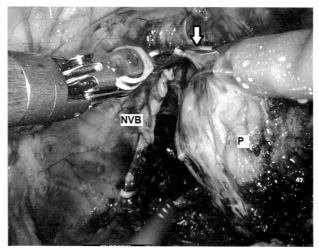

Figure 11.23 Nerve sparing. Dissection of the levator and prostatic fascia, containing the NVB, off the prostate (P) using cold scissors is continued until the left puboprostatic ligament (arrow).

- Bleeding from the dilated periprostatic veins may occur. It usually stops spontaneously, avoiding unnecessary electrocautery.

The same steps are followed for the other side.

- The dissection can be continued posterior to the prostate through the same plane toward the level of prostatic apex distally (Figure 11.24).

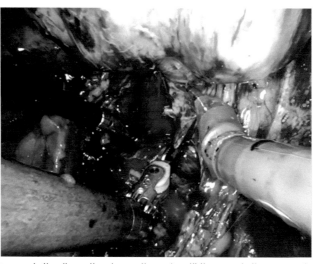

Figure 11.24 Posterior prostatic dissection is continued until the prostatic apex releasing the urethroprostatic attachment.

DVC AND URETHRAL DIVISION

- The intra-abdominal pressure is increased to 20 mmHg to prevent significant bleeding during division of DVC.
- The DVC is transected just proximal to the apex level using hot shears until the urethra is reached (Figure 11.25).
- The assistant provides irrigation and limited suction to blood and fluid to avoid dropping the intra-abdominal pressure causing more bleeding.
- The urethra is divided by cold scissors and the urethral catheter is partially withdrawn by the second assistant to complete the urethral transection (Figure 11.26).
- Posteriorly a small apical prostatic lip may be encountered extending distally.

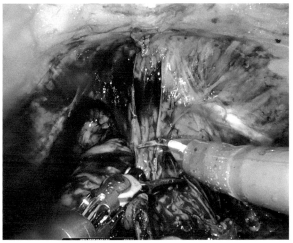

Figure 11.25 DVC transection.

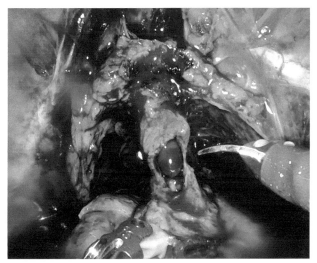

Figure 11.26 Sharp transection of the urethra by cold scissors.

Avoiding positive margin at the apex should not significantly compromise the urethral length.

- Rectaurethralis and remaining Denonvilliers' fascia attachment are gently and carefully released.

> Rectal tenting during removal of the prostate due to posterior apical attachment keeps the rectum at risk of injury.

- The excised prostate and the previously resected prostatic fat are introduced into an endo-catch bag.
- The bag is closed and the thread is clipped to ensure the closure.

HEMOSTASIS AND DVC SUTURING

- A temporary compression on DVC is applied by the ProGrasp on a cotton gauze.
- Meanwhile the dissection area at the prostatic bed and Denonvilliers' fascia above the rectum is cleaned by suction irrigation.
- Active bleeding, if present, is secured by clips, suturing or by selective bipolar coagulation and a hemostatic agent such as FloSeal is applied (Figure 11.27).

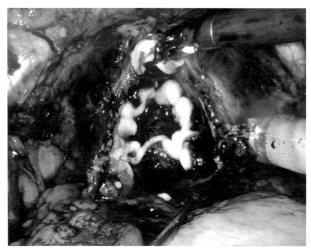

Figure 11.27 Hemostasis. Application of Flo on the prostatic bed with cotton gauze pressure on DVC.

Pelvic lymph node dissection (PLND) if indicated is performed at this step.

- The arm 1 and 3 instruments are changed to needle drivers.
- The DVC is closed by continuous running suturing using a 15-cm, 3/0 V-Loc stitch on a 17 mm, 1/2 circle, CV-23 needle.
- Suturing is performed from left to right and the remaining stitch can be utilized for later right side anterior reconstruction.
- The intra-abdominal pressure is reduced back to 12 mmHg after this step, the FloSeal is washed out and hemostasis is reassessed (Figure 11.28).

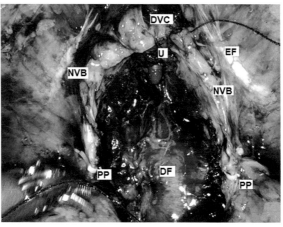

Figure 11.28 Prostatic bed. *Abbreviations*: DF, Denonvilliers' fascia; DVC, deep vascular complex; EF, left endopelvic fascia; NVB, neurovascular bundles; PP, clipped prostatic pedicles; U, urethra.

POSTERIOR RECONSTRUCTION (MODIFIED ROCCO STITCH)

- Posterior reconstruction incorporates the longitudinal muscles of posterior bladder neck and Denonvilliers' fascia to the periurethral tissue of rectourethralis muscle (Figure 11.29).
- Suturing is performed by using a 15-cm, 3/0 V-Loc stitch on a 17-mm 1/2 circle, CV-23 needle, from left to right, cephalo-caudal direction in three running stitches.

> The posterior reconstruction provides a tension-free vesicourethral anastomosis and may enhance early recovery of post-prostatectomy incontinence.

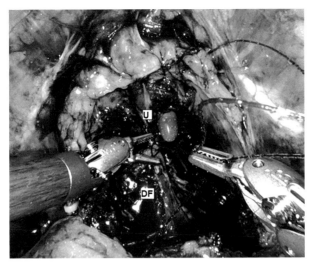

Figure 11.29 Posterior reconstruction. DF, Denonvilliers' fascia; U, urethra.

VESICOURETHRAL ANASTOMOSIS

Visual field orientation is essential to achieve accurate anastomosis. Camera rotation is avoided and the symphysis pubis is always positioned at 12 o'clock.

- The anastomosis begins at 5 o'clock position, using the same V-Loc stitch of the posterior reconstruction which ended just right to the urethra (Figure 11.30).

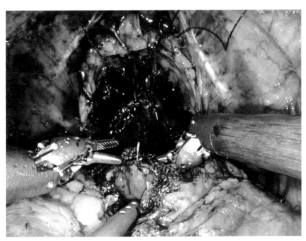

Figure 11.30 Vesicourethral anastomosis starting at 5 o'clock on the bladder neck. Suction probe down traction exposes posterior bladder neck.

- The anastomosis is performed by continuous running suturing starting first on the left side then on the right.

Throughout the anastomosis, the suturing is always outside-in at the bladder and inside-out at the urethra.

For every urethral stitch, the second assistant should manipulate the catheter tip in/out to open the urethra and guide the surgeon's needle (Figure 11.31).

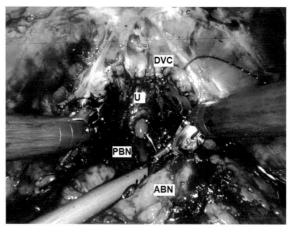

Figure 11.31 The needle is guided by the Foley catheter. *Abbreviations*: ABN, anterior bladder neck; DVC, sutured deep vascular complex; PBN, posterior bladder neck; U, urethra.

- After making the bladder neck 6 o'clock stitch, the suture line is tightened, approximating the bladder to the urethra.

For left side precise suturing from 7 to 11 o'clock:

- The bladder outside-in is performed by the left hand.
- The urethral inside-out is performed by the right hand (Figure 11.32).

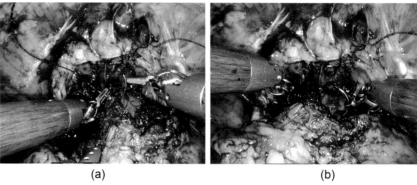

| (a) | (b) |

Figure 11.32 Left side (7–11 o'clock) vesicourethral anastomosis. (a) Outside-in at the bladder neck by left hand. (b) Inside-out at the urethra by right hand.

Everting the bladder mucosa is not a must; however, including a few millimeters from mucosal edge is crucial and sufficient to ensure a mucosa to mucosa anastomosis.

- With suction device, the assistant exposes the bladder neck wall and clears the field and urethra from blood.
- Once the left side anastomosis reaches 11 o'clock, a similar V-Loc 3/0 stitch is introduced to start suturing the right side from 4 o'clock to 12 o'clock.

For right side precise suturing from 4 to 12 o'clock:

- The bladder outside-in is performed by the right hand.
- The urethral inside-out is performed by the left hand (Figure 11.33).

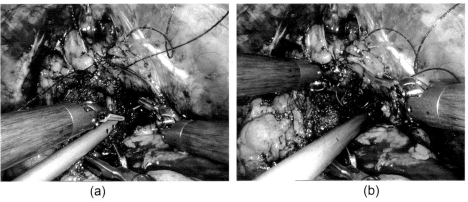

(a)   (b)

Figure 11.33 Right side (4–12 o'clock) vesicourethral anastomosis. (a) Outside-in at the bladder neck by right hand. (b) Inside-out at the urethra by left hand.

> To avoid tearing of the urethral wall while tightening the anastomosis line, the stitch is pulled straight perpendicular to the wall, which can be further supported by the other hand instrument (Figure 11.34).

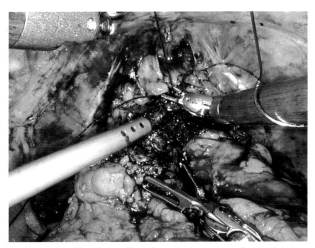

Figure 11.34 Tightening the suture line by pulling the stitch perpendicular to the urethral wall, supported by the left-hand needle driver. *Abbreviations*: BN, bladder neck; U, urethra.

- The residual anterior bladder neck gap is closed by the remaining right side anastomosis stitch before tying it with the left one.
- Another V-Loc stitch may be required if the bladder neck gap is quiet large.

During this step, the second assistant should make sure that the urethral catheter is not entrapped by the stitch and is moving freely in and out.

- The catheter is replaced by a new one because it may have been injured during needle guiding.
- The anastomosis integrity is assessed by filling the bladder to 150 mL of normal saline looking for fluid leakage. Unrecognized bladder wall injury or residual gaps can also be identified.

ANTERIOR RECONSTRUCTION

- Detrusor muscle and perivesical fat around the bladder neck is continuously sutured to the levator fascia and puboprostatic ligaments.
- On the right side, this can be performed by utilizing the remaining stitch used for DVC closure.
- A sling stitch for the bladder neck to the symphysis pubis is performed (Figure 11.35).

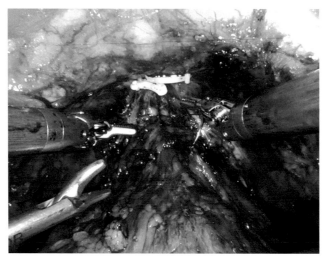

Figure 11.35 Sling stitch from the bladder neck to the pubic bone.

HEMOSTASIS, WOUND CLOSURE, DRAIN AND SPECIMEN EXTRACTION

- Hemostatic agent such as Surgicel may be placed at sides of the bladder neck if necessary.
- Drain is inserted through a lateral 8-mm port wound.
- Wounds of >10 mm are closed using a Carter Thomason device.

A detailed explanation of drain and closure along with figures are provided in Section 1.

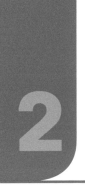

Transperitoneal Robot-Assisted Laparoscopic Partial Nephrectomy

POSITION

- The patient is positioned in a semi-lateral (60°) decubitus position with the abdomen at the table edge (Figure 12.1).
- Straps, adhesives and supporting pads are applied to stabilize the patient, and the urinary catheter is inserted before the draping.

The table is not flexed in a transperitoneal approach to avoid unnecessary rhabdomyolysis and postoperative neuromusculoskeletal pain.

Table flexion may also decrease the working space by pushing the kidney close to the abdominal wall.

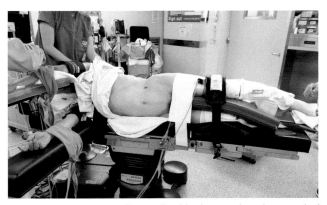

Figure 12.1 Semi-lateral decubitus position. The patient is strapped and supported; shoulder and pressure areas are padded; electrocautery is connected; urethral catheter is inserted; intermittent pneumatic calf compression device and elastic stocking are applied.

ACCESS

- In the lateral decubitus position, the Veress needle is introduced through a 1.5-cm ipsilateral hemi-circumferential incision around the umbilicus (Figure 12.2).

Confirmation of Veress needle passage and position is explained in Chapter 3, Section 1 "Basic Instrumentation".

Access

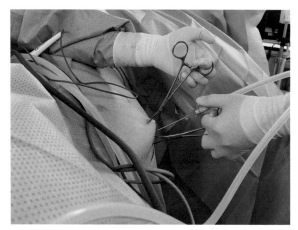

Figure 12.2 Veress needle insertion in lateral position. The abdominal wall is stabilized by two towel clips.

- Gas flow can be increased once Veress needle correct position is confirmed and 1 L is insufflated.
- Pneumoperitoneum is created to 15 mmHg for trocar insertion, after which it is set down to 12 mmHg throughout the procedure.

Access can also be obtained by open (Hasson) technique or under direct vision using optiview trocar with the laparoscope (Chapter 6, Figure 6.3).

FIRST PORT INSERTION

- A 12-mm disposable trocar is inserted at the access site.
- A da Vinci Xi 30° lens laparoscope is introduced to assess:

  - Veress needle and port entry area for any injury
  - Operation site and kidney outline
  - Presence of adhesions
  - Entry sites of the next port
  - Survey for abnormal anatomy or lesions

ROBOTIC TROCAR INSERTION AND DOCKING OF THE ROBOT

- Three or four 8-mm robotic port sites are marked on the skin and the trocars are inserted (Figure 12.3).
- For the right kidney, a 5-mm liver retraction trocar is inserted just inferior to the xiphoid process.

One assistant 12-mm umbilical port is usually enough, and if an additional one is required, it can be inserted at midline, supra- or infra-umbilicus.

- The robotic cart is allocated to the back of the patient.
- The camera is docked for targeting and repositioning of the robotic arms before docking the other ports.

THE ROBOTIC FOUR ARM INSTRUMENTS

  - Maryland Bipolar Forceps, Fenestrated (left hand)
  - Camera: 30°
  - Hot shear monopolar curved scissors (right hand)
  - ProGrasp forceps

Access site and number (three or four arms) and configuration of port placement may vary depending on the tumor side, size, location, kidney anatomy, the patient body habitus and surgeon's preference.

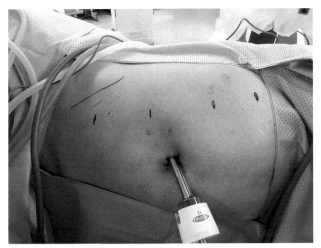

Figure 12.3 The four arms, robotic port site configurations for left-side partial nephrectomy with the 12-mm assistant disposable trocar at the umbilicus.

ASSISTING SURGEONS AND OPERATING ROOM SETUP

- *Position:* At the patient's abdominal side, using the 12-mm ports.
- *Role:* Retraction, suction of blood and gas, changing robotic arms, cleaning the camera, applying clips and Bulldog vascular clamps, introducing and taking out instruments, needles and supplies.
- The operating room is set up to facilitate a smooth flow of surgery (Figure 12.4).

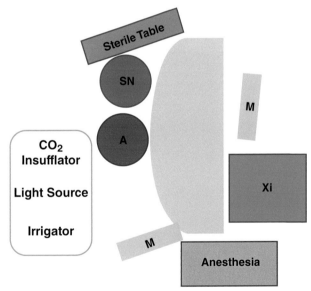

Figure 12.4 Diagram of the operation room setup showing the surgical team positions in relation to the patient, monitors (M), robotic cart (Xi) and the accessory machines. *Abbreviations*: A, assistant surgeon; SN, scrub nurse.

STEP-BY-STEP SURGERY

ADHESIOLYSIS AND LIVER RETRACTION

- Adhesiolysis is performed if significant bowel adhesions are present at operation area or at port's entry sites.
- In the right side, the liver and gallbladder adhesions are released before introducing the retractor. The triangular ligament may need to be divided at this step.

171

- The liver retraction trocar is inserted just inferior to the xiphoid process.

To avoid liver injury while inserting the retraction port, a right angle can be applied against the anterior abdominal wall around the entry point of the trocar (Figure 12.5).

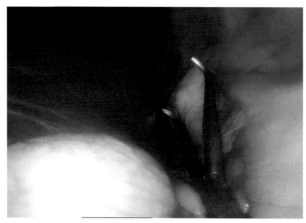

Figure 12.5 Using a right-angled clamp against anterior abdominal wall during insertion of the 5-mm liver retraction trocar to avoid liver injury.

- Atraumatic non-crushing locking grasper is introduced and fixed to the diaphragm muscles supero-laterally (Figure 12.6).

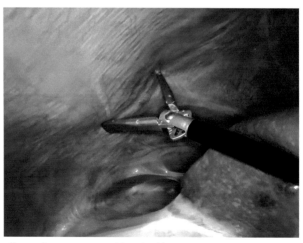

Figure 12.6 Liver retraction using a non-crushing locking grasper.

COLON (DESCENDING OR ASCENDING) MOBILIZATION

- The peritoneum is opened at the white line of Toldt just lateral to the colon, and the bowel is reflected medially.
- A plane between the white perinephric fat of Gerota and the yellow fat of the mesocolon is created by blunt and sharp dissection (Figure 12.7).

Meticulous and careful use of the cautery at this step is mandatory to avoid injuries to the colon or its mesentery.

- The dissection is carried out from the level of common iliac vessels inferiorly up to the level of the colonic flexure and/or the diaphragm superiorly at the upper pole.

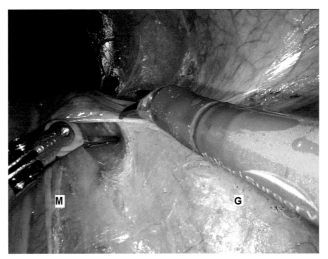

Figure 12.7 The peritoneum is opened at the white line of Toldt. Dissection is performed in avascular plane between the white perinephric fat of Gerota (G) and the yellow fat of mesocolon (M).

> The planes are opened carefully from superficial to deep, layer by layer, up and down along the line of dissection.
> Injuries or bleeding in deep and narrow spaces are difficult to manage due to inadequate exposure.

Dissecting the lateral Gerota attachment at this step must be avoided. That will drop down the kidney medially and make the hilar dissection difficult.

> Oncologic surgery should be embryologic surgery. If the dissection is performed between the embryologically different planes, it should be easy and oncologically safe. Being an avascular plane, the bleeding should be minimal.

IN THE RIGHT SIDE

- The hepatorenal and posterior coronary ligaments are incised and extended to the diaphragm if complete kidney mobilization is required (Figure 12.8).

> The division of hepatorenal and posterior coronary ligaments will expose the lateral wall of vena cava above the adrenal gland, duodenum and renal hilum.

- After reflecting the colon medially, the duodenum is defined and Kocherized to reveal the anterior surface of the inferior vena cava (IVC) (Figure 12.9).

Close contact to the duodenum by cautery must be avoided.

IN THE LEFT SIDE

- The usual extensive colon mobilization and upper pole dissection may not be necessary in partial nephrectomy unless complete mobilization of the kidney is required depending on tumor size or location.
- The splenocolic, linorenal and phrenicocolic ligaments are carefully incised (Figure 12.10).

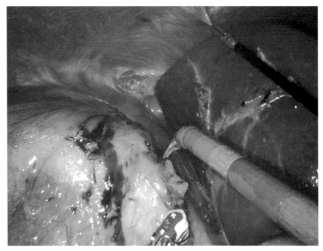

Figure 12.8 Hepatorenal ligament incision.

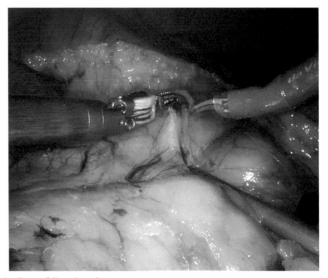

Figure 12.9 Kocherization of the duodenum.

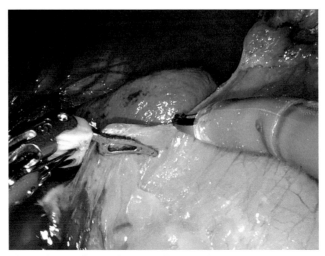

Figure 12.10 Incising the splenocolic and linorenal ligaments.

Once the linorenal and splenocolic ligaments are divided, the spleen, pancreas and colon will drop and reflect medially.

This decreases the risk of injury, during later dissection of the hilum, adrenal gland and upper pole.

Take care to avoid spleen and stomach injury if extensive dissection of the left upper pole attachment is performed.

- The tail of pancreas is further released from the adrenal gland and upper pole of the kidney, taking care to avoid injury to the pancreatic tissue or the splenic vessels.

PSOAS MUSCLE, URETER AND GONADAL VESSELS

Ureteric and gonadal dissection and isolation may not be necessary unless kidney mobilization is required or in case of lower pole tumor.

- Inferiorly, the anterior layer of Gerota's fascia is opened and dissected just lateral to IVC in the right side or to aorta on the left.
- The gonadal vein and ureter are identified in the fibrofatty tissue above the psoas muscle.
- They are dissected and released from the psoas muscle, together with the surrounding fat.
- The inferior Gerota's fascia with the ureter-gonadal vein packet is retracted anterolaterally by the ProGrasp or the assistant retractor exposing the psoas muscle (Figure 12.11).

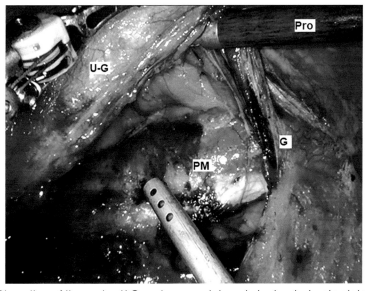

Figure 12.11 Dissection of the ureter: U-G, ureter-gonadal packet retracted anterolaterally by ProGrasp (Pro). *Abbreviations*: G, medial Gerota attachment; PM, psoas muscle.

The anterolateral retraction of ureter-gonadal vein packet will stretch the medial and the posterior Gerota attachment and will facilitate the dissection.

Take care to avoid excessive traction to prevent renal arterial spasm or right gonadal vein avulsion injury at the level of the IVC.

POSTEROMEDIAL DISSECTION

- Once the kidney is on traction, the posterior surface of Gerota's fascia will be clearly visualized.
- The posterior areolar attachment of Gerota to the psoas muscle is freed by blunt and sharp dissection (Figure 12.12).

Psoas fascia should be released intact to avoid muscle fiber exposure and unwanted bleeding.

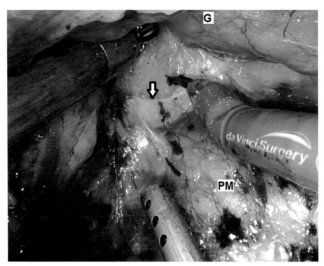

Figure 12.12 Posterior dissection. *Abbreviations*: G, posterior Gerota; PM, psoas muscle. Psoas fascia (arrow).

- The anteromedial Gerota attachment is released superficially layer by layer to avoid injuries to the gonadal vein or crossing vessels to the kidney and ureter (Figure 12.13).

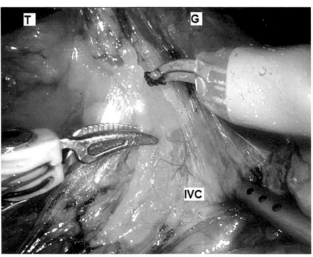

Figure 12.13 Sharp release of stretched anteromedial Gerota attachment. *Abbreviations*: G, anterior Gerota's fascia; IVC, inferior vena cava; T, anterolateral traction.

- In the right side, the gonadal vein may be seen joining the IVC. It can be clipped and divided to avoid traction injury and significant bleeding (Figure 12.14).
- The fibro-lymphovascular tissue at the hilum around the pedicle is dissected superficially and with caution to prevent inadvertent vascular injuries.
- The bulky tissue attachment or small vascular branches can be clipped and/or transected by monopolar scissors.

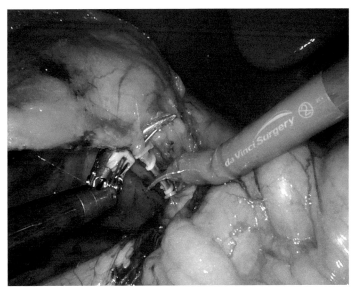

Figure 12.14 Right gonadal vein.

Applying multiple clips around the pedicle should be avoided. They may interfere with vascular clamping particularly in case of emergency.

THE PEDICLE

In the left side, the colon may fall back laterally on the field; it can be retracted by a stitch using suture passer needle through the abdominal wall.

- Once the Gerota attachment is cleared, the renal vein can be clearly identified under mild tension because of gentle traction.

The vena cava in the right and gonadal vein in the left can be used as guidance landmarks to the renal vein.

- The ProGrasp is repositioned to be just at the lower pole of the kidney providing better exposure with a gentle stretch of the pedicle.

If complete kidney mobilization is not indicated, then the pedicle can be approached directly through the hilum without extensive inferior or superior dissection.

- The anterior and inferior surfaces of the renal vein are cleared from fibrofatty tissue (Figure 12.15).
- The left gonadal vein may need to be clipped at this level if interfering with this step.
- A lumbar vein joining the left renal vein may be identified. It is isolated, clipped by Hem-o-lok and divided (Figure 12.16).

If the lumbar vein is not well controlled or injured during dissection, it may retract into the muscle and will be hard to catch and control.

Division of the left gonadal and lumbar vein will expose the renal artery.

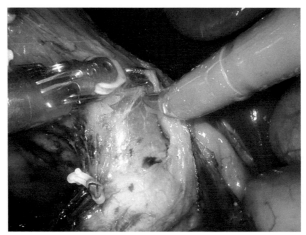

Figure 12.15 Dissection of right renal vein. Gonadal vein is seen clipped on IVC.

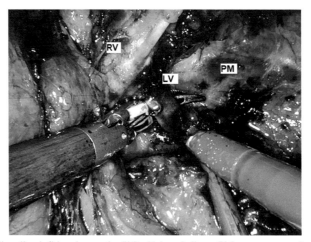

Figure 12.16 Dissecting the left lumbar vein (LV). *Abbreviations*: PM, psoas muscle; RV, left renal vein.

- The tissue posterior to the vein is carefully dissected looking for the renal artery which can be recognized by its pulsation or as a white tubular structure (Figure 12.17).
- The periarterial tissue attachment is dissected by Maryland and coagulated and transected away from the vessel by monopolar scissors (Figure 12.18).

Complete arterial skeletonization from the perivascular adventitia is not necessary.

- The artery is circumferentially freed and isolated on a vessel loop (Figure 12.19).

> To avoid excessive bleeding surprise during resection, reviewing the preoperative imaging study to assess for early branching artery and to rule out multiple or accessory arteries is crucial.

- If required, the renal vein can be further dissected circumferentially and an adequate window is created.
- A vessel loop is placed around the vein and the loop is clipped.

> The vessel loop is utilized to manipulate the vessel for accurate clamping. It also provides an easy, safe and fast approach in case of emergency or severe bleeding.

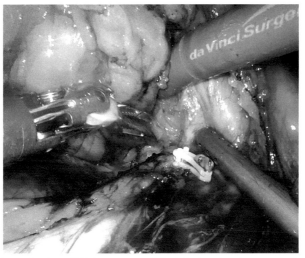

Figure 12.17 The right renal artery (RA) is seen as white tubular structure posterior to the renal vein.

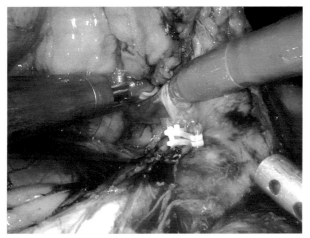

Figure 12.18 The periarterial lymphovasular tissue is dissected gently by Maryland and transected using monopolar diathermy away from the vessel.

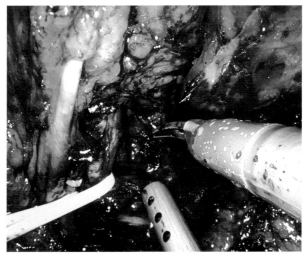

Figure 12.19 The left renal artery is isolated on a vessel loop.

ADRENAL GLAND

- In case of upper pole tumor or whole kidney mobilization is required, the adrenal gland is dissected and separated.
- The Gerota's fascia is opened just above the renal vein and the perinephric fat is dissected upward immediately on the anteromedial surface of renal parenchyma.
- The adrenal gland is separated from the upper pole of the kidney by blunt and sharp dissection using electrocautery.

Take care to avoid injuries to aberrant vessels or other structures such as pancreas, IVC and aorta medially.

TUMOR DISSECTION

> For precise tumor resection and to avoid positive margins, excessive bleeding or long ischemia time, it is crucial for the tumor to be circumferentially accessible.

- Once the tumor area is localized with or without kidney mobilization, the Gerota's fascia is opened near the tumor location on the normal parenchyma.
- The perinephric fat is cleared off the parenchyma for at least 1 cm beyond the tumor edge (Figure 12.20).

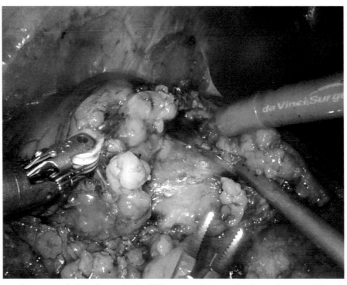

Figure 12.20 The perinephric fat is dissected off the renal capsule 1 cm beyond the tumor margins and resection line is marked by cautery. The fat on the tumor is preserved.

- If possible, it is better not to remove the fat covering the tumor as it can be used to grasp and manipulate the mass during dissection.

If the tumor is endophytic or its limit is undetermined, an intraoperative ultrasound introduced through the assistant port can be utilized.

PEDICLE CLAMPING

- Once the tumor area is prepared and kidney position is adjusted for easy access around the tumor, mannitol and frusemide can be given 15 minutes before pedicle clamping as reno-protectants.
- The line of resection is marked by cautery on the normal parenchyma capsule keeping about 5 mm of safe margin around the tumor.

To provide further kidney stabilization to achieve an optimal angle for easy tumor resection and renorrhaphy, the Gerota's fascia can be retracted to the abdominal wall by a PDS or nylon stitch using a Carter Thomason needle.

- The artery is retracted by the vessel loop to open a safe window for a Bulldog vascular clamp (Figure 12.21).

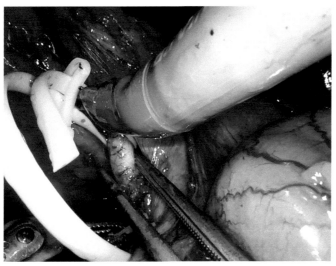

Figure 12.21 Pedicle clamping.

Take care to be steady when the assistant introduces the Bulldog clamp to avoid poking the vessels or going further inside blindly.

The console surgeon should instruct and direct the assistant for correct clamp positioning by providing a satisfactory visual field and a wide clear window around the artery.

- The warm ischemia time is set once the artery is clamped.

If the main artery is clamped, the vein should collapse, if not then look for another artery.

Clamping the vein is usually not necessary unless the tumor is large or central or has got a sizable vein seen on preoperative images. This may provide a bloodless field during tumor resection and renal construction.

TUMOR RESECTION

- The marked parenchyma around the tumor is incised circumferentially and superficially using cold scissors (Figure 12.22).
- The curve of the scissors is directed downward and away from the tumor to facilitate the resection of the tumor to accurate depth and width.

Using electrocautery for resection may obscure the demarcation of normal tumor tissue and can alter the histological structure.

- The ProGrasp or the assistant grasper stabilizes the kidney while the left-hand Maryland gently countertracts the mass to expose the resection line.

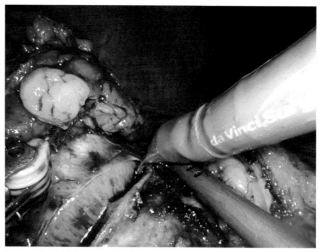

Figure 12.22 Tumor is resected at the marked parenchyma directing the scissors downward. The mass is retracted by the left-hand Maryland. The assistant applies a gentle countertraction on the kidney by suction probe.

- The tumor violation during resection must be avoided, and the resection line exposure can be achieved by manipulating the tumor fat or by gentle back traction using the other hand instrument.
- The assistant should apply gentle parenchymal pressure in addition to continuous suction-irrigation of blood to improve the visualization of resection line.

> Irrigation is preferred over suction to clear the field of vision, as excessive suction reduces the intraperitoneal pressure, causing bothersome back bleeding.

Keeping a gauze piece in the field for hemostasis may be necessary if significant bleeding is anticipated.

- The incision is deepened by sharp and blunt dissection all around toward the base of tumor (Figure 12.23).

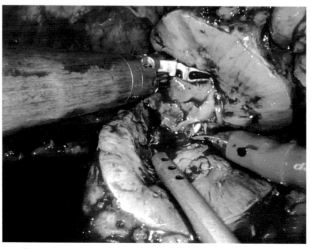

Figure 12.23 Resection of the tumor base. The assistant provides suction-irrigation and applies a gentle downward traction.

- Once the deepest portionv of the tumor is incised, the scissors' curve is directed upward.
- Active arterial bleeder can be controlled during or after tumor resection using a small size clip (Figure 12.24).

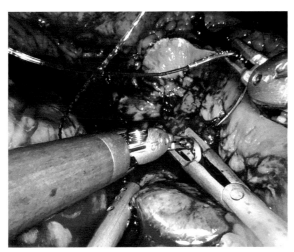

Figure 12.24 Active arterial bleeder is clipped after tumor resection.

- Once the tumor is completely excised, it is placed into an endo-catch bag which is closed, secured by Hem-o-lok and left aside.

RENAL RECONSTRUCTION

- The resection bed is oversewn using a 23-cm, 3/0 V-Loc absorbable stitch on 1/2 circle of (26 mm) V-20 needle.
- The stitch is inserted through the renal capsule at the distal end of the wound.

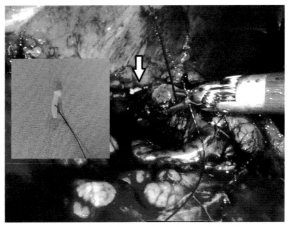

Figure 12.25 An anchoring Hem-o-lok clip at the end of V-Loc stitch will ensure a tense suturing without cutting through the parenchyma (arrow).

Step-by-Step Surgery

- The needle is introduced just deep enough to include part of the cortex, medulla and pelvicalyceal system together in a continuous running suturing (Figure 12.26).

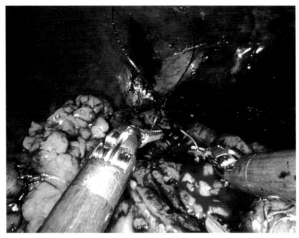

Figure 12.26 Renal bed reconstruction using V-Loc stitch.

- At the stitch exit of the wound, a clip is applied on the renal capsule, maximizing the tension of the suture line (Figure 12.27).

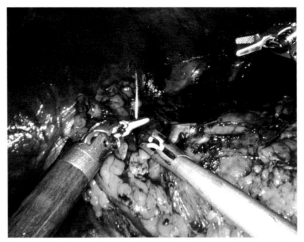

Figure 12.27 The renal reconstruction suture line is tightened by applying a clip at the V-Loc stitch exit on the renal capsule.

- If the resection area is large, then two or more stitches are used, dividing the bed into two or more parts.

Careful renal tissue handling and slow meticulous suturing are mandatory to avoid tissue laceration or bleeding, leading to a long ischemia time.

- The Bulldog clamps are carefully removed by the assistant, making sure the jaws are opened well enough to avoid significant vascular injuries.

Early pedicle unclamping approach will reduce the ischemia time and facilitate identifying active bleeding for better control.

The vein clamps are removed before the arterial ones.

- The resection area is inspected for active bleeding.
- A second layer renorrhaphy is performed using a 33-cm, 3/0 PDS stitch on 1/2 circle, 31-mm, MH-1 needle.

> In hilar masses, the tumor bed reconstruction is carefully performed to avoid vascular injuries or ligation and renorrhaphy may not always be possible.

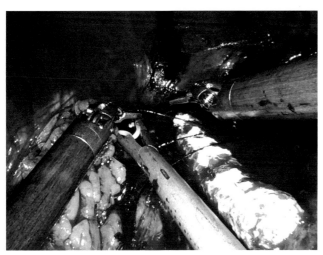

Figure 12.28 Renorrhaphy over TachoSil hemostatic agent and suture lines are tightened by Hem-o-lok clips.

- The renal defect is closed by approximating the parenchyma over a TachoSil roll (bolster) (Figure 12.28).
- The suture lines are tightened by placing Hem-o-lok clips at each side of the stitches on the renal capsule.

> A second layer (renorrhaphy) may not be necessary if there is no significant bleeding or urine leak after renal pedicle unclamping, particularly in small defects.
>
> Tumor bed suturing and application of a hemostatic agent such as tissue glue or Surgicel should be adequate.

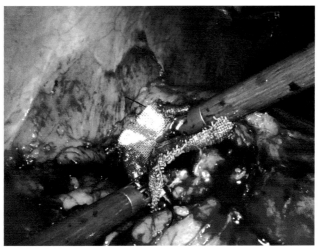

Figure 12.29 A wound clotting agent is applied over the renal wound gap.

- A hemostatic agent or perinephric fat can be utilized to cover the suture line or residual gap if present (Figure 12.29).

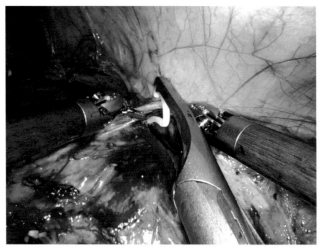

Figure 12.30 Nephropexy.

- If the kidney was completely mobilized, then nephropexy is performed. The Gerota's fascia is clipped to the lateral peritoneal reflection on the lateral abdominal wall by Hem-o-lok clips (Figure 12.30).

SPECIMEN RETRIEVAL, DRAIN INSERTION AND WOUND CLOSURE

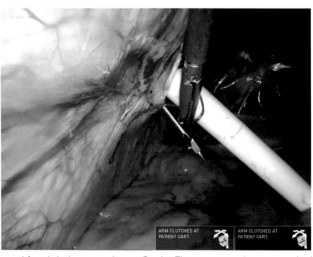

Figure 12.31 Port wound fascial closure using a Carter Thomason suture pass device.

- The specimen is removed through the assistant port site or through a Gibson incision if large.
- A drain is inserted and the fascia of wounds more than 10 mm are closed by using a Carter Thomason suture pass device on 1/0 vicryl stitch (Figure 12.31).

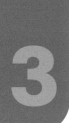

Retroperitoneal Robot-Assisted Laparoscopic Partial Nephrectomy

- The preferred tumor sites for retroperitoneal over transperitoneal approach are illustrated in (Figure 13.1).

Transperitoneal approach is preferred over retroperitoneal in complex cases of endophytic, large tumors (>4 cm), hilar location and presence of huge perinephric fat or as a surgeon's preference.

POSITION

- The patient is positioned in a complete lateral decubitus (90°) position with the abdomen at the table edge.
- Table is flexed at level of the umbilicus (Figure 13.2).
- Straps, adhesives and supporting pads are applied to stabilize the patient, and the urinary catheter is inserted before the draping.

Flexing the table at full lateral decubitus position increases the working space by increasing the distance between the costal margin and iliac crest and the distance between the quadratus lumborum and colon.

ACCESS AND FIRST TROCAR INSERTION

- The retroperitoneal access is achieved by open technique in the lateral position.
- A 2-cm incision around 2 cm superior and medial to anterior-superior iliac spine (ASIS) is made (Figure 13.3).

The access site may differ depending on the tumor site, kidney anatomy and surgeon's preference and experience.

- The wound is deepened by muscle splitting using a straight hemostat directing it perpendicular to the patient axis until the retroperitoneal fat is seen.

The wound layer exposure and separation is achieved by S retractors and the aid of the laparoscopic bright light if required.

DOI: 10.1201/b22928-16

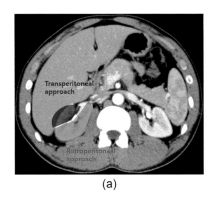

(a)

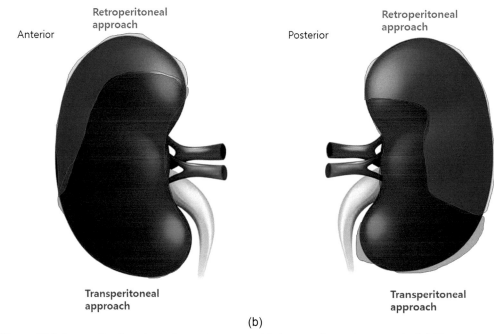

Anterior

Retroperitoneal
approach

Transperitoneal
approach

Posterior

Retroperitoneal
approach

Transperitoneal
approach

(b)

Figure 13.1 Tumor sites for retroperitoneal compared to transperitoneal approach. (a) Contrast-enhanced axial sections CT scan. (b) Diagram of anterior and posterior kidney surfaces.

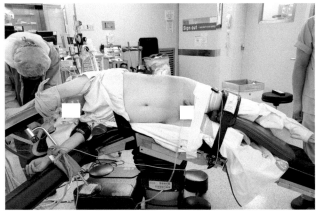

Figure 13.2 Complete lateral (90°) position with table flexion at the umbilicus. The patient is strapped and supported; shoulder and pressure areas are padded; electrocautery is connected; urethral catheter is inserted; intermittent pneumatic calf compression device and elastic stocking are applied.

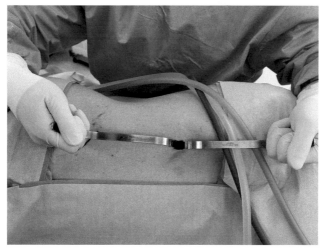

Figure 13.3 Retroperitoneal access. A 2-cm wound, 2 cm above and medial to the ASIS. Fascial layers are exposed by S retractors.

- A wet index finger is introduced into the retroperitoneum and a space is created.
- Finger dissection is performed by gentle sweeping movement between the psoas muscle posteriorly and the Gerota's fascia and peritoneal reflection anteriorly.

> To prevent peritoneal injury while accessing the retroperitoneal space, directing the hemostat or finger dissection anteromedially must be avoided.

- Once a maximum space is achieved, a balloon dilator is inserted parallel to psoas muscle and directed cranially (Figure 13.4).
- The balloon is inflated by around 400 mL of air (35–40 pumps), and an obvious tense localized distension is observed.
- Balloon dilatation can also be performed under a direct vision with the laparoscope inside the trocar.

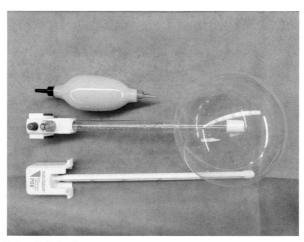

Figure 13.4 Balloon dilator (inflated).

Keeping the balloon inflated for a couple of minutes may provide a local retroperitoneal hemostasis.

- A disposable 12-mm port at this site is usually quite adequate to prevent air leak during surgery. If gas seal is not optimal, the wound gap can be closed by silk stitch.
- Gas is insufflated through this port and pneumoretroperitoneum is created to minimum of 12 mmHg.

- A da Vinci Xi, 30° lens laparoscope is introduced to assess:

  - Active bleeding due to access or balloon dissection
  - Peritoneum for any injuries
  - Gerota's fascia with kidney and psoas muscle outline
  - The entry sites of next trocars

ROBOTIC TROCAR INSERTION

- Three da Vinci Xi 8-mm robotic trocars are inserted at or just cephalad to the midway between the iliac crest and costal margins (Figure 13.5):

  - *Camera port*: Mid-axillary line
  - *Right and left robotic ports*: Anterior and posterior axillary

- The distance between the instruments is around 6 cm.

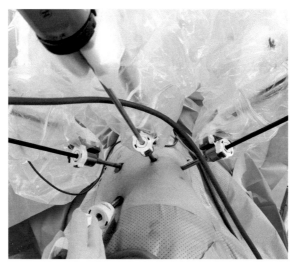

Figure 13.5 Trocar configurations for left partial nephrectomy.

The port sites may differ depending on the tumor site, kidney anatomy and surgeon's preference and experience.

- To ensure a safe trocar entry, if required, the posterolateral fat and the anteromedial peritoneum can be dissected off the abdominal wall using a suction probe or monopolar scissors (Figure 13.6).

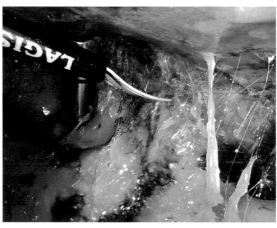

Figure 13.6 Clearing off the abdominal wall fat at the secondary trocar entry sites before insertion.

ASSISTING SURGEON AND THE ROBOTIC INSTRUMENTS

- Assistant position: At the patient's abdominal side, using the access (12 mm) port.

  - *Role*: Retraction, suction of blood and gas, changing robotic arms, cleaning the camera, applying clips and Bulldog vascular clamps, introducing and taking out instruments, needles and supplies

- The robotic instruments:

  - Maryland bipolar forceps, fenestrated (left hand)
  - Camera: 30° lens
  - Hot shear monopolar curved scissors (right hand)

- The operating room is set up to facilitate a smooth flow of surgery (Figure 13.7).

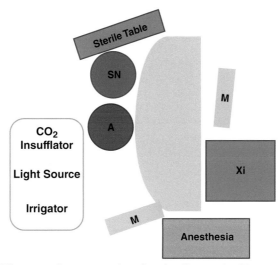

Figure 13.7 Diagram of the operation room setup showing the surgical team positions in relation to the patient, monitors (M), robotic cart (Xi) and the accessory machines. *Abbreviations*: A, assistant surgeon; SN, scrub nurse.

STEP-BY-STEP SURGERY

GEROTA'S FASCIA DISSECTION

- The retroperitoneal paranephric fat is dissected off the Gerota's fascia and psoas muscle (Figure 13.8).

> The narrow working space and the anatomic limitations with no clear landmarks are the main challenges of retroperitoneal approach.
> The psoas muscle is the key for orientation and should always be in a longitudinal horizontal view.

- Careful and meticulous dissection is continued on the psoas muscle toward the kidney without violating the psoas fascia.
- The Gerota's fascia is opened as far possible posteromedially to avoid incising the peritoneum.
- The psoas muscle will be clearly visualized posteriorly and the Gerota's incision is widened parallel to the muscle (Figure 13.9).
- The perinephric fat is dissected toward the hilum aiming for the pedicle.
- Retracting the kidney anteromedially by the assistant retractor will further expose the dissection plane and keeps the hilum stretched.

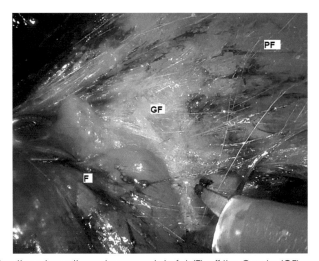

Figure 13.8 Dissecting the retroperitoneal paranephric fat (F) off the Gerota (GF) and psoas fascia (PF).

If the peritoneum is perforated, the gas will leak to the peritoneal cavity and may compromise the retroperitoneal space. Three ways to overcome this situation:

1. Suturing or clipping of the peritoneal gap.
2. Retraction with fan retractor through an additional trocar to minimize the leak.
3. Enlarge the peritoneal incision.

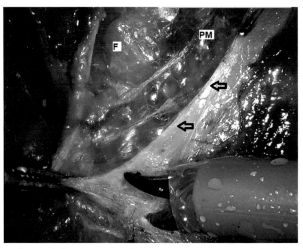

Figure 13.9 Incising the Gerota's fascia (arrows). *Abbreviations*: F, perinephric fat; PM, psoas muscle.

Dissecting deep medially may injure the vena cava and duodenum on the right side, or the aorta and superior mesenteric artery on the left.

- If difficulty is encountered finding the pedicle, the dissection is carried out inferiorly looking for the lower pole and ureter.
- The ureter can be identified as a longitudinal white tubular structure with peristalsis parallel to the psoas muscle leading to the hilum.

The ureter and gonadal vein are not dissected if kidney mobilization is not required.

HILAR DISSECTION

Anatomical orientation when dealing with the pedicle is crucial to avoid mistaking the renal vessels with other vessels or vital structures.

- At the hilum, the renal artery can be recognized by its pulsation over the fat or seen as a vertically oriented tubular structure (Figure 13.10).
- The artery is circumferentially dissected from its periarterial neurolymphatic tissue and isolated.
- In left side, the lumbar vein may be encountered while dissecting for the artery. If it is interfering with the pedicle dissection, it can be clipped using Hem-o-lok and divided in-between.
- The perivascular tissue is coagulated and transected away from the arterial wall by the right-hand monopolar scissors (Figure 13.11).

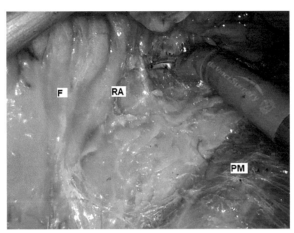

Figure 13.10 Hilar dissection. RA (renal artery) is oriented vertically. *Abbreviations*: F, perinephric fat; PM, psoas muscle.

Complete arterial skeletonization from the perivascular adventitia is not necessary.

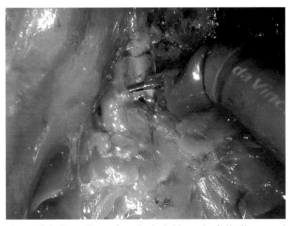

Figure 13.11 Gentle and careful dissection of periarterial lymphofatty tissue using right-hand monopolar scissors.

- The artery is isolated and encircled vessel loop and the loop is clipped by Hem-o-lok (Figure 13.12).

> Reviewing the preoperative imaging study is critical to assess for early branching artery and to rule out multiple or accessory arteries.

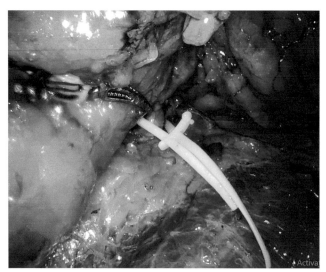

Figure 13.12 Isolation of renal artery on a vessel loop.

- The renal vein is usually seen anterior and inferior to the artery. If required, it is dissected and circumferentially freed, creating an adequate window and is encircled by a vessel loop.

> The vessel loop is utilized to manipulate the vessel for accurate clamping. It also provides an easy, safe and fast approach in case of emergency and severe bleeding.

- The left adrenal and gonadal veins may also be identified. They can be saved if the renal vein is adequately isolated.

TUMOR DISSECTION

The renal pedicle at the hilum is used as a landmark for kidney orientation and tumor localization.

- The perinephric fat is cleared off the parenchyma around 1 cm beyond the tumor edge.
- It is better not to remove the fat covering the tumor if possible. The fat can be used to grasp and manipulate the mass during dissection.

> For precise tumor resection and to avoid positive margins, excessive bleeding or long ischemia time, it is crucial for the tumor to be circumferentially accessible.

- Further Gerota's fascia dissection requiring kidney mobilization may occasionally be necessary depending on the tumor size and location.

Due to its limitations, patient selection for retroperitoneal approach is important to avoid extensive anterior kidney dissection.

> The perinephric fat and/or the peritoneum may fall on the dissection field. They can be retracted to anterior abdominal wall by a 3/0 stitch using a Carter Thomason needle.

If the tumor is endophytic or its limit is undetermined, an intraoperative ultrasound introduced through the assistant port can be utilized.

PEDICLE CLAMPING

- Once tumor area is prepared and kidney position is optimized for accurate resection and suturing, frusemide and mannitol can be given 15 minutes before pedicle clamping as reno-protectant.
- The line of resection is marked by cautery on the normal parenchyma capsule keeping about 5 mm of safe margin around the tumor (Figure 13.13).
- The artery is retracted by the vessel loop to open a safe window for the Bulldog vascular clamp (Figure 13.14).

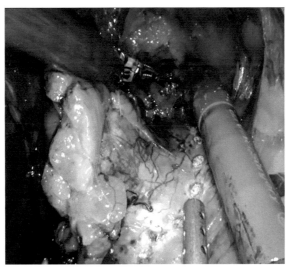

Figure 13.13 The perinephric fat is dissected off the renal capsule 1 cm beyond the tumor margins. The tumor fat is preserved and the resection line is marked by cautery.

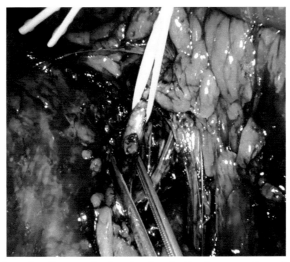

Figure 13.14 Pedicel clamping. The renal artery is retracted by the vessel loop for safe and accurate application of the Bulldog vascular clamp by the assistant.

Take care to be steady when the assistant introduces the Bulldog clamp to avoid poking the vessels or going further inside blindly.

The console surgeon should instruct and direct the assistant for proper clamp positioning by providing a satisfactory visual field and a wide clear window around the artery.

- The warm ischemia time is set once the artery is clamped.

If the main artery is clamped, the vein should collapse, if not then look for another artery.

> Clamping the vein is usually not necessary unless the tumor is large or central or has a sizable vein seen on preoperative image. This may provide a bloodless field during tumor resection and renal construction.

TUMOR RESECTION

- The marked parenchyma around the tumor is incised circumferentially and superficially using cold scissors (Figure 13.15).
- The curve of the scissors is directed downward and away from the tumor to facilitate the resection of the tumor to accurate depth and width.

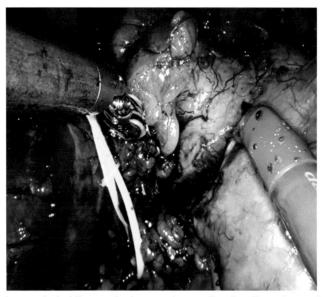

Figure 13.15 Tumor is resected at the marked parenchyma directing the scissors downward. The mass is retracted by the left-hand Maryland.

Using electrocautery for tumor resection may obscure the demarcation of normal tumor tissue and can alter the histological structure.

- The left-hand Maryland gently countertracts and manipulates the mass by the fat on the tumor or by grasping the resected collecting system.

Keeping a gauze piece in the field for hemostatsis may be necessary if significant bleeding is anticipated.

- The assistant should apply gentle parenchymal pressure in addition to continuous suction-irrigation of blood to improve the visualization of resection line.

> Irrigation is preferred to clear the field of vision as excessive suction quickly reduces the retroperitoneal pressure, collapsing the work space and causing bothersome back bleeding.

- The incision is deepened by sharp and blunt dissection all around toward the base of the tumor (Figure 13.16).

- Once the deepest part of the tumor is incised, the scissor curve is directed upward.

> Reviewing the preoperative images to evaluate the tumor size, depth and configuration is crucial.

- Active arterial bleeder during resection can be clipped using small size clip.
- Once the tumor is completely excised, it is placed into an endo-catch bag which is closed and secured by a Hem-o-lok clip and left aside.

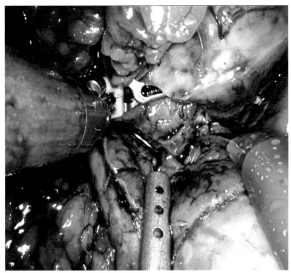

Figure 13.16 Resection of the tumor base. The assistant provides suction-irrigation and applies a gentle downward traction.

RENAL RECONSTRUCTION

- The resection bed is over-sewn using a 23 cm, 3/0 V-Loc absorbable stitch on 1/2 circle of (26 mm) V-20 needle.
- The stitch is inserted through the renal capsule at the distal end of the wound.

A Hem-o-lok clip at the tail end of the stitch will ensure tense suturing without cutting through the parenchyma (Figure 13.17).

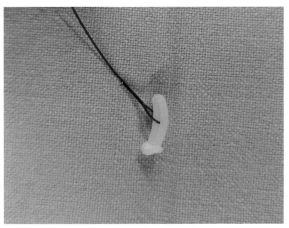

Figure 13.17 An anchoring Hem-o-lok clip at the end of V-Loc stitch.

- The needle is introduced just deep enough to include part of the cortex, medulla and pelvicalyceal system together in a continuous running suturing (Figure 13.18).

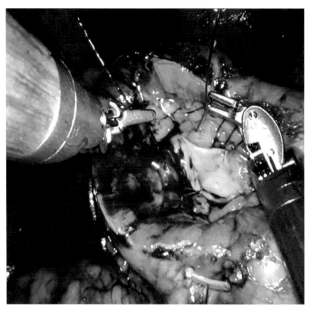

Figure 13.18 Renal bed reconstruction using V-Loc stitch. Note the open calyces.

- At the stitch exit of the wound, a clip is applied on the renal capsule, maximizing the tension of the suture line (Figure 13.19).

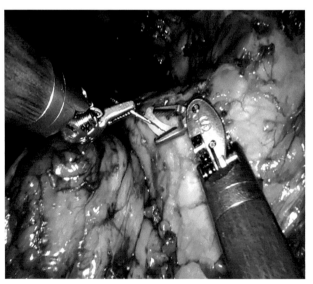

Figure 13.19 The renal reconstruction suture line is tightened by a clip at the stitch exit on the renal capsule.

- If the resection area is large, then two or more stitches are used, dividing the bed into two or more parts.

Take care of renal tissue handling and use slow meticulous suturing, which is mandatory to avoid tissue laceration or bleeding, leading to long ischemia time.

- The Bulldog clamps are removed carefully by the assistant making sure that the jaws are opened well enough to avoid significant injuries.

The vein clamps are removed before the arterial ones.

> Early pedicle unclamping approach will reduce the ischemia time and will facilitate identifying active bleeding for better control.

- The resection area is inspected for active bleeding.
- A second layer renorrhaphy is performed using a 33-cm, 3/0 PDS stitch on 1/2 circle (31 mm), MH-1 needle.
- The renal defect is closed by approximating the parenchyma over a TachoSil roll (bolster) (Figure 13.20).

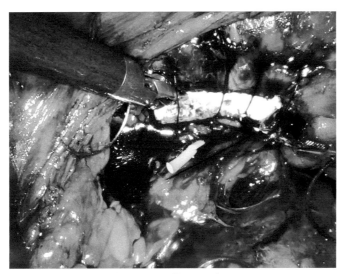

Figure 13.20 Renorrhaphy over a TachoSil hemostatic agent.

- The suture line is tightened by placing Hem-o-lok clips at each side of stitches on the renal capsule (Figure 13.21).

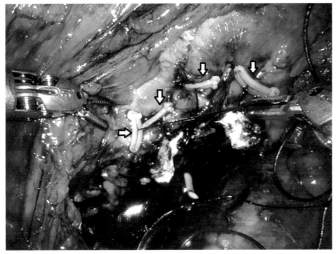

Figure 13.21 The renorrhaphy suture lines are tightened by placing Hem-o-lok clips (arrows) at each side of the stitches on the renal capsule.

- A hemostatic agent or perinephric fat can be utilized to cover the suture line or the residual gap if present (Figure 13.22).

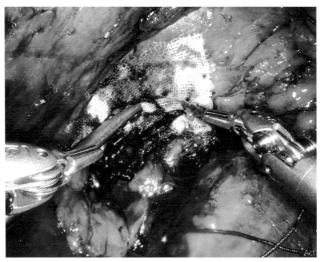

Figure 13.22 A wound clotting agent is applied on the renal wound.

A second layer (renorrhaphy) may not be necessary if there is no significant bleeding or urine leak after renal pedicle unclamping, particularly in small defects.

Tumor bed suturing and application of hemostatic agent such as tissue glue or Surgicel should be adequate.

SPECIMEN RETRIEVAL, DRAIN INSERTION AND WOUND CLOSURE

- The specimen is removed through the assistant port (access) site which can be extended in case of large tumors.
- A drain is inserted and the access wound is closed in layers.

Retroperitoneal Robotic Partial Nephrectomy

Bibliography

Allaf ME, Bhayani SB, Rogers C, et al. Laparoscopic partial nephrectomy: evaluation of long term oncological outcome. *J Urol* 2004;172:871–873.

Bhayani SB, Rha KH, Pinto PA, et al. Laparoscopic partial nephrectomy: effect of warm ischemia on serum creatinine. *J Urol* 2004;172:1264–1266.

Badani KK, Kaul S, Menon M. Evolution of robotic radical prostatectomy: assessment after 2766 procedures. *Cancer* 2007;110:1951–1958.

Berguer R. Surgical technology and the ergonomics of laparoscopic instruments. *Surg Endosc.* 1998;12:458–462.

Berguer R, Gerber S, Klipatrick G, Remler M, Beckley DA. Comparison of forearm and thumb muscle electromyographic responses to the use of laparoscopic instruments with either a finger grasp or a palm grasp. *Ergonomics* 1999;42:1634–1645.

Berguer R, Rab G, Abu-Ghaida H, Alarcon A, Chung J. A comparison of surgeons' posture during laparoscopic and open surgical procedures. *Surg Endosc* 1997;11:139–142.

Berguer R, Forkey DL, Smith WD. The effect of laparoscopic instrument working angle on surgeons' upper extremity workload. *Surg Endosc* 2001;15:1027–1039.

Berguer R, Smith WD, Davis S. An ergonomic study of the optimum operating table height for laparoscopic surgery. *Surg Endosc* 2002;16:416–421.

Berryhill R Jr, Jhaveri J, Yadav R, et al. Robotic prostatectomy: a review of outcomes compared with laparoscopic and open approaches. *Urology* 2008;72(1):15–23.

Blom JH, van Poppel H, Marechal JM, et al. Radical nephrectomy with and without lymph-node dissection: final results of European Organization for Research and Treatment of Cancer (EORTC) randomized phase 3 trial 30881. *Eur Urol* 2009;55:28–34.

Breda A, Stepanian SV. Use of haemostatic agents and glues during laparoscopic partial nephrectomy: a multi-institutional survey from the United States and Europe of 1347 cases. *Eur Urol* 2007;52(3):798–803.

Brennan TA, Leape LL, Laird NM, et al. Incidence of adverse events and negligence in hospitalized patients. Results of the Harvard Medical Practice Study I. *N Engl J Med* 1991;324:370–376.

Busby JE, Matin SF. Laparoscopic radical nephroureterectomy for transitional cell carcinoma: where are we in 2007? *Curr Opin Urol* 2007;17(2):83–87.

Cadeddu JA, Wolfe JS Jr, Nakada SY, et al. Complications of laparoscopic procedures after concentrated training in urological laparoscopy. *J Urol* 2001;166(6):2109–2111.

Chan D, Bishoff JT, Ratner L, et al. Endovascular gastrointestinal stapler device malfunction during laparoscopic nephrectomy: early recognition and management. *J Urol* 2000;164:319–321.

Chang SL, Kibel AS, Brooks JD, Chung BI. The impact of robotic surgery on the surgical management of prostate cancer in the USA. *BJU Int* 2015;115:929–936.

Chiu A, Azadzoi K, Hatzichristou DG, et al. Effects of intra-abdominal pressure on renal tissue perfusion during laparoscopy. *J Endourol* 1994;8:99–103.

Chiu AW, Chen KK, Wang JH, Huang WJ, Chang LS. Direct needle insufflation for pneumoretroperitoneum: anatomic confirmation and clinical experience. *Urology* 1995;46:432–437.

Clayman RV, Kavoussi LR, Soper NJ, et al. Laparoscopic nephrectomy: initial case report. *J Urol* 1991; 146:278–282.

Clayman RV, Kavoussi LR, Soper NJ et al. Laparoscopic nephroureterectomy: initial case report. *J Laparoendosc Surg* 1991;1:343–349.

Costello AJ, Brooks M, Cole OJ. Anatomical studies of the neurovascular bundle and cavernosal nerves. *BJU Int* 2004;94:1071–1076.

de la Rosette JJ, Gill IS. *Laparoscopic Urologic Surgery in Malignancies.* Springer, Berlin, Heidelberg, New York, 2005.

Eden CG, Coptcoat MJ. Assessment of alternative tissue approximation techniques for laparoscopy. *Br J Urol* 1996;78:234–242.

Erdogru T, Teber D, Frede T, et al. Comparison of transperitoneal and extraperitoneal laparoscopic radical prostatectomy using match-pair analysis. *Eur Urol* 2004;46(3):312–319.

Fahlenkamp D, Rassweiler J, Fornara P, Frede T, Loening SA. Complications of laparoscopic procedures in urology: experience with 2,407 procedures at 4 German centers. *J Urol* 1999;162:765–770.

Ficarra V, Novara G, Artibani W, et al. Retropubic, laparoscopic, and robotassisted radical prostatectomy: a systematic review and cumulative analysis of comparative studies. *Eur Urol* 2009;55:1037–1063.

Finelli A, Gill IS. Laparoscopic partial nephrectomy: contemporary technique and results. *Urol Oncol* 2004;22:139–144.

Florio G, Silvestro C, Polito DS. Periumbilical veress needle pneumoperitoneum: technique and results. *Chir Ital* 2003;55:51–54.

Frede T, Stock C, Renner C, et al. Geometry of laparoscopic suturing and knotting techniques. *J Endourol* 1999;13(3):191–198.

Galanakis I, Vasdev N, Soomro N. A review of current hemostatic agents and tissue sealants used in laparoscopic partial nephrectomy. *Rev Urol* 2011;13:131–138.

Gaur DD. Laparoscopic operative retroperitoneoscopy: use of a new device. *J Urol* 1992; 148:1137–1139.

Hanna GB, Shimi S, Cuschieri A. Optimal port locations for laparoscopic intracorporeal knotting. *Surg Endosc* 1997;11:397–401.

Gill IS, Kavoussi LR, Lane BR, et al. Comparison of 1,800 laparoscopic and open partial nephrectomies for single renal tumors. *J Urol* 2007;178:41–46.

Gill IS, Rassweiler JJ. Retroperitoneoscopic renal surgery: our approach. *Urology* 1999;54:734–738.

Gill IS, Sung GT. Laparoscopic radical nephroureterectomy for upper tract transitional cell carcinoma: the Cleveland Clinic experience. *J Urol* 2000;164(5):1513–1522.

Guillonneau B, Jayet C, Tewari A, Vallancien G. Robot assisted laparoscopic nephrectomy. *J Urol* 2001;166:200–201.

Guillotreau J, Game X, Mouzin M, et al. Radical cystectomy for bladder cancer: morbidity of laparoscopic versus open surgery. *J Urol* 2009;181:554–549.

Hacker A, Albadour A. Nephron-sparing surgery for renal tumours: acceleration and facilitation of the laparoscopic technique. *Eur Urol* 2007;51(2):358–365.

Hafez KS, Fergany AF, Novick AC. Nephron sparing surgery for localized renal cell carcinoma: impact of tumor size on patient survival, tumor recurrence and TNM staging. *J Urol* 1999;162: 1930–1933.

Hamade AM, Butt I. Closed blunt-trocar 5 mm-port for primary cannulation in laparoscopic surgery: a safe technique. *Surg Laparosc Endosc Percutan Tech* 2006;16(3):156–160.

Hanna GB, Shimi SM, Cuschieri A. Task performance in endoscopic surgery is influenced by location of the image display. *Ann Surg* 1998;227:481–484.

Hasson HM. A modified instrument and method for laparoscopy. *Am J Obstet Gynecol* 1971; 110:886–887.

Hemal AK, Kumar A. Laparoscopic versus open radical nephrectomy for large renal tumors: a long-term prospective comparison. *J Urol* 2007; 177(3):862–866.

Hemal AK, Srinivas M, Charles AR. Ergonomic problems associated with laparoscopy. *J Endourol.* 2001;15:499–503.

Horgan S, Vanuno D. Robots in laparoscopic surgery. *J Laparoendosc Adv Surg Tech A* 2001;11:415–419.

Jackson MR, Taher MM, Burge JR, et al. Hemostatic efficacy of a fibrin sealant dressing in an animal model of kidney injury. *J Trauma* 1998;45:662–665.

Johnston 3rd WK, Wolf Jr JS. Laparoscopic partial nephrectomy: technique, oncologic efficacy, and safety. *Curr Urol Rep* 2005;6:19–28.

Kowalczyk KJ, Levy JM, Caplan CF, et al. Temporal national trends of minimally invasive and retropubic radical prostatectomy outcomes from 2003 to 2007: results from the 100% Medicare sample. *Eur Urol* 2012;61:803–809.

Landman J, Kerbl K, Rehman J, et al. Evaluation of a vessel sealing system, bipolar electrosurgery, harmonic scalpel, titanium clips, endoscopic gastrointestinal anastomosis vascular staples and sutures for arterial and venous ligation in a porcine model. *J Urol* 2003;169(2):697–700.

Lane BR, Gill IS. Seven-year oncological outcomes after laparoscopic and open partial nephrectomy. *J Urol* 2010;183:473–479.

Li WM, Shen JT, Li CC, et al. Oncologic outcomes following three different approaches to the distal ureter and bladder cuff in nephroureterectomy for primary upper urinary tract urothelial carcinoma. *Eur Urol* 2010;57:963–969.

Link RE, Su L-M, Sullivan W, et al. Health related quality of life before and after laparoscopic radical prostatectomy. *J Urol* 2005;173:175–179.

Lotan Y, Cadeddu JA, Gettman MT. The new economics of radical prostatectomy: cost comparison of open, laparoscopic and robot assisted techniques. *J Urol* 2004;172:1431–1435.

Liu CD, McFadden DW. Laparoscopic port sites do not require fascial closure when nonbladed trocars are used. *Am Surg* 2000;66(9):853–854.

Liu JJ, Maxwell BG, Panousis P, Chung BI. Perioperative outcomes for laparoscopic and robotic compared with open prostatectomy using the National Surgical Quality Improvement Program (NSQIP) database. *Urology* 2013;82:579–583.

Liu ZW, Olweny EO, Yin G, et al. Prediction of perioperative outcomes following minimally invasive partial nephrectomy: role of the RENAL nephrometry score. *World J Urol* 2013;31:1183–1189.

Manasnayakorn S, Cuschieri A, Hanna GB. Ideal manipulation angle and instrument length in hand-assisted laparoscopic surgery. *Surg Endosc* 2008;22:924–929.

Mattar K, Finelli A. Expanding the indications for laparoscopic radical nephrectomy. *Curr Opin Urol* 2007;17(2):88–92.

Matern U. The laparoscopic surgeon's posture, In: S.M. Bogner, ed., *Misadventures in Health Care: Inside Stories*, Lawrence Erlbaum Assosiates, Inc., Mahwah, NJ, London, 2003.

Matern U, Faist M, Kehl K, Giebmeyer C, Buess G, Monitor position in laparoscopic surgery. *Surg Endosc* 2005;19:436–440.

Mattern U, Waller P. Instruments for minimally invasive surgery: principles of ergonomic handles. *Surg Endosc* 1999;13:174–182.

Matern U, Waller P, Giebmeyer C, Rückauer KD, Farthmann EH. Ergonomics: requirements for adjusting the height of laparoscopic operating tables. *J Soc Laparoendosc Surg* 2001;5:7–12.

Menon M, Kaul S, Bhandari A, et al. Potency following robotic radical prostatectomy: a questionnaire based analysis of outcomes after conventional nerve-sparing and prostatic fascia-sparing techniques. *J Urol* 2005;174:2291–2296.

Menon M, Muhletaler F, Campos M, et al. Assessment of early continence after reconstruction of the periprostatic tissues in patients undergoing computer-assisted (robotic) prostatectomy: results of a 2 group parallel randomized controlled trial. *J Urol* 2008;180(3):1018–1023.

Miller DC, Saigal CS, Banerjee M, et al. Diffusion of surgical innovation among patients with kidney cancer. *Cancer* 2008;112:1708–1717.

Ng CK, Kauffman EC, Lee MM, et al. A comparison of postoperative complications in open vs robotic cystectomy. *Eur Urol* 2010;57:274–281.

Ni S, Tao W, Chen Q, et al. Laparoscopic versus open nephroureterectomy for the treatment of upper urinary tract urothelial carcinoma: a systematic review and cumulative analysis of comparative studies. *Eur Urol* 2012;61:1142–1153.

Ong AM, Su LM, Varkarakis I, et al. Nerve sparing radical prostatectomy: effects of hemostatic energy sources on the recovery of cavernous nerve function in a canine model. *J Urol* 2004;172(4 Pt. 1):1318–1322.

Ono Y, Hattori R. Laparoscopic radical nephrectomy for renal cell carcinoma: the standard of care already? *Curr Opin Urol* 2005;15(2):75–78.

Orvieto MA, Chien GW, Laven B, et al. Eliminating knot tying during warm ischemia time for laparoscopic partial nephrectomy. *J Urol* 2004;172(6 Pt. 1):2292–2295.

Orvieto MA, Lotan T, Lyon MB, et al. Assessment of the LapraTy clip for facilitating reconstructive laparoscopic surgery in a porcine model. *Urology* 2007;69(3):582–585.

Oz MC, Rondinone JF, Shargill NS. FloSeal Matrix: new generation topical hemostatic sealant. *J Card Surg* 2003;18:486–493.

Parra RO, Andrus CH, Jones JP et al. Laparoscopic cystectomy: initial report on a new treatment for retained bladder. *J Urol* 1992;148:1140–1144.

Parsons JK, Varkarakis I, Rha KH, et al. Complications of abdominal urologic laparoscopy: longitudinal five-year analysis. *Urology* 2004;63:27–32.

Patel HD, Mullins JK, Pierorazio PM, et al. Trends in renal surgery: robotic technology is associated with increased use of partial nephrectomy. *J Urol* 2013;189:1229–1235.

Patel VR, Palmer KJ, Coughlin G, Samavedi S. Robot-assisted laparoscopic radical prostatectomy: perioperative outcomes of 1500 cases. *J Endourol* 2008;22:2299–2305.

Pérez-Duarte FJ, Sánchez-Margallo FM, Díaz-Güemes I, Sánchez-Hurtado MA, Lucas-Hernández M, Usón Gargallo J. Ergonomics in laparoscopic surgery and its importance in surgical training. *Cir Esp* 2011;90:284–289.

Permpongkosol S, Link RE. Complications of 2,775 urological laparoscopic procedures: 1993 to 2005. *J Urol* 2007;177(2):580–585.

Philips PA, Amaral JF. Abdominal access complications in laparoscopic surgery. *J Am Coll Surg* 2001; 19:525–536.

Odeberg-Wernerman S. Laparoscopic surgery – effects on circulatory and respiratory physiology: an overview. *Eur J Surg Suppl* 2000;585:4–11.

Ponsky L, Cherullo E, Moinzadeh A, et al. The Hem-o-lok clip is safe for laparoscopic nephrectomy: a multi-institutional review. *Urology* 2008;71(4):593–596.

Pruthi RS, Wallen EM. Robotic assisted laparoscopic radical cystoprostatectomy: operative and pathological outcomes. *J Urol* 2007;178:814–818.

Ramani AP, Desai MM, Steinberg AP, et al. Complications of laparoscopic partial nephrectomy in 200 cases. *J Urol* 2005;173:42–47.

Rambourg P, Saint-Remy JM, Sturm C, Watson N. Evaluating the differences between fibrin sealants: recommendations from an international advisory panel of hospital pharmacists. *Eur J Hosp Pharm Sci* 2006;12(1):3–9.

Rassweiler JJ, Schulze M. Laparoscopic nephroureterectomy for upper urinary tract transitional cell carcinoma: is it better than open surgery? *Eur Urol* 2004; 46(6):690–697.

Rassweiler J, Tsivian A, Kumar AV, et al. Oncologic safety of laparoscopic surgery for urological malignancy: experience with more than 1,000 operations. *J Urol* 2003;169:2072–2075.

Reddy, PP, Reddy TP, Roig-Francoli J, et al. The impact of the Alexander technique on improving posture and surgical ergonomics during minimally invasive surgery: pilot study. *J Urol* 2011;186(4):1658–1662.

Richstone L, Montag S, Ost MC, et al. Predictors of hemorrhage after laparoscopic partial nephrectomy. *Urology* 2011;77:88–91.

Rocco B, Gregori A, Stener S, et al. Posterior reconstruction of the rhabdosphincter allows a rapid recovery of continence after transperitoneal videolaparoscopic radical prostatectomy. *Eur Urol* 2007;51(4):996–1003.

Rocco F, Carmignani L, Acquati P, et al. Restoration of posterior aspect of rhabdosphincter shortens continence time after radical retropubic prostatectomy. *J Urol* 2006;175(6):2201–2206.

Rocco F, Carmignani L, Acquati P, et al. Early continence recovery after open radical prostatectomy with restoration of the posterior aspect of the rhabdosphincter. *Eur Urol* 2007;52(2):376–383.

Romero FR, Muntener M. Pure laparoscopic radical nephrectomy with level II vena caval thrombectomy. *Urology* 2006;68(5):1112–1114.

Roupret M, Hupertan V. Oncologic control after open or laparoscopic nephroureterectomy for upper urinary tract transitional cell carcinoma: a single center experience. *Urology* 2007;69(4):656–661.

Saber AA, Meslemani AM. Safety zones for anterior abdominal wall entry during laparoscopy: a CT scan mapping of epigastric vessels. *Ann Surg* 2004;239(2):182–185.

Scheussler WW, Schulam PG, Clayman RV et al. Laparoscopic radical prostatectomy: initial short term experience. *Urology* 1997;50:854–857.

Scosyrev E, Messing EM, Sylvester R, et al. Renal function after nephron-sparing surgery versus radical nephrectomy: results from EORTC randomized trial 30904. *Eur Urol* 2014;65:372–377.

Shalhav AL, Barret E. Transperitoneal laparoscopic renal surgery using blunt 12-mm trocar without fascial closure. *J Endourol* 2002;16(1):43–46.

Shalhav AL, Orvieto MA, Chien GW, et al. Minimizing knot tying during reconstructive laparoscopic urology. *Urology* 2006;68(3):508–513.

Simone G, Papalia R, Guaglianone S, et al. Laparoscopic versus open nephroureterectomy: perioperative and oncologic outcomes from a randomized prospective study. *Eur Urol* 2009;56:520–526.

Smith AK, Lane BR, Larson BT, et al. Does the choice of technique for management of the bladder cuff affect oncologic outcomes of nephroureterectomy for upper tract urothelial cancer? *J Urol* 2009;181:133–134.

Stephenson AJ, Gill IS. Laparoscopic radical cystectomy for muscle-invasive bladder cancer: pathological and oncological outcomes. *BJU Int* 2008;102:1296–1301.

Stifelman MD, Caruso RP, Nieder AM, Taneja SS. Robot-assisted laparoscopic partial nephrectomy. *JSLS* 2005;9:83–86.

Stroup SP, Palazzi K, Kopp RP, et al. RENAL nephrometry score is associated with operative approach for partial nephrectomy and urine leak. *Urology* 2012;80:151–156.

Studer UE, Burckard FC, Schumacher M, et al. Twenty years experience with an ileal orthotopic low pressure bladder substitute–lessons to be learned. *J Urol* 2006;176:161–166.

Szeto G, Cheng S, Poon J, Ting A, Tsang R, Ho P. Surgeons' static posture and movement repetitions in open and laparoscopic surgery. *J Surg Res* 2012, 172(1):e19–e31.

Van Det MJ, Meijerink WJ, Hoff C, et al. Optimal ergonomics for laparoscopic surgery in minimally invasive surgery suites: a review and guidelines. *Surg Endosc* 2009;23:1279–1285.

Van Dijk JH, Pes PL. Haemostasis in laparoscopic partial nephrectomy: current status. *Minim Invasive Ther Allied Technol* 2007;16(1):31–44.

Van Poppel H, Da Pozzo L, Albrecht W, et al. A prospective randomized EORTC intergroup phase 3 study comparing the complications of elective nephronsparing surgery and radical nephrectomy for low-stage renal cell carcinoma. *Eur Urol* 2007;51:1606–1615.

Van Veelen MA, Kazemier G, Koopmann J, Goossens RHM, Meijer DW. Assessment of the ergonomically optimal work surface height for laparoscopic surgery. *J Laparoendosc Adv Surg Tech A* 2002;12(1):47–52.

Van Veelen MA, Meiier DW. Ergnomics and design of laparoscopic instruments: results of a survey among laparoscopic surgeons. *J Laparoendosc Adv Surg Tech A* 1999;9:481–489.

Van Veelen MA, Nederlof EAL, Goossens RHM, Schot CJ, Jakimowicz JJ. Ergonomic problems encountered by the medical team related to products used for minimally invasive surgery. *Surg Endosc* 2003;17:1077–1081.

Verhoest G, Manunta A. Laparoscopic partial nephrectomy with clamping of the renal parenchyma: initial experience. *Eur Urol* 2007;52(5):1340–1346.

Wang GJ, Barocas DA, Raman JD, Scherr DS. Robotic vs. open radical cystectomy: prospective comparison of perioperative outcomes and pathological measures of early oncological efficacy. *BJU Int* 2007;101:89–93.

Wauben LS, Albayrak A, Goossens RHM. Ergonomics in the operating room – an overview, In: Brinkerhoff BN, ed., *Ergonomics: Design, Integration, and Implementation*, Nova Science Publishers, New York, 2009:79–118.

Wolf JS, Stoller M. The physiology of laparoscopy: basic principles, complications and other considerations. *J Urol* 1994;152:294–302.

Zehetner J, Kaltenbacher A, Wayand W, Shamiyeh A. Screen height as an ergonomic factor in laparoscopic surgery. *Surg Endosc* 2006;20:139–141.

Index

Note: *Italic* page numbers refer to figures.

access
  entry and exit 19–20, *19–20*
  laparoscopic partial nephrectomy 89–90, *89–91*
  laparoscopic radical nephrectomy 51–52, *52*
  laparoscopic radical nephroureterectomy 69–70, *70*
  open (Hasson) technique 20
  retroperitoneal laparoscopic nephrectomy 109–111, *110–111*
  retroperitoneal robotic partial nephrectomy 187, *189*, 189–190
  robotic partial nephrectomy 169–170, *170, 171*
  veress needle *19,* 19–20, *20*
adhesiolysis 53, *54–55*
adrenalectomy
  laparoscopic radical nephrectomy 66
  laparoscopic radical nephroureterectomy 84
adrenal gland preservation
  laparoscopic radical nephrectomy 65–66, *66*
  laparoscopic radical nephroureterectomy 82–83, *82–83*
  retroperitoneal laparoscopic nephrectomy 117, *117*
angles
  elevation *24,* 24
  manipulation 11, *12, 24,* 24
  suturing 11, *12*
  working 4, *4,* 24
anterior superior iliac spine (ASIS) 109
assistant surgeon positions, robotic radical prostatectomy 151, *151*
atraumatic locking grasper 8, *9*

Babcock forceps 8
balloon dilator 21, *21*

balloon trocar 23, *24*
baseball diamond concept 24, *24*
bladder cuff excision 85–87, *85–87*
bladder neck dissection 39–41, *39–41,* 156–158, *157–158*
bladder pedicle control, laparoscopic radical cystoprostatectomy 131–132, *131–132*
bolster 15, *16,* 185, 199
Bulldog vascular clamp, applicator 12, *13*
bunching stitch 37, 39

camera (laparoscope) 8
Carter Thomason suture pass device 25, *25, 49, 67,* 87, 186, *186*
cellulose polymer 15
clips and clip applicators *13,* 13–14, *14*
colon mobilization
  laparoscopic partial nephrectomy *93,* 93–94, *94*
  laparoscopic radical nephrectomy 55–56, *55–56*
  laparoscopic radical nephroureterectomy 73–74, *73–74*
  robotic partial nephrectomy 172–173, *173*
cystostomy 11, 86, *87*

da Vinci Xi robotic cart 7, 21
decubitus position 51, 69, 89, 109, 169, *169,* 187
Denonvilliers' fascia 43–45, *43, 46,* 125, *126,* 132, 134, 159, 160, *161,* 161, 163, *164, 165*
diamond-shaped configuration 59, *59*
dorsal vascular complex (DVC) 156
drains 16, *17*
  Jackson-Pratt 16, *17*
  laparoscopic partial nephrectomy 108

drains (*cont.*)
    laparoscopic radical cystoprostatectomy
       135, *136*
    laparoscopic radical nephrectomy 67, *67*
    laparoscopic radical nephroureterectomy 87
    laparoscopic radical prostatectomy 49
    retroperitoneal laparoscopic nephrectomy 117
    retroperitoneal robotic partial
       nephrectomy 200
    robotic partial nephrectomy 186, *186*
    robotic radical prostatectomy 168
DVC *see* dorsal vascular complex

endopelvic fascia 34–37, *34–35*, *39*, 128–130,
    128–129, *154*, 155–156, *157*, *164*
energy devices 7, 36, 39, 55, 66, 78, 115, 132
    electrocautery/ultrasonic machines 7
entry and exit
    access 19–20, *19–20*
    balloon dilator 21, *21*
    balloon trocar 23, *24*
    port configuration 24–25, *24–25*
    port site closure 25, *25*
    trocar insertions *22*, 22–23, *23*
    trocars 21, *21*, *22*
ergonomics in laparoscopy 3

fan retractor 10, *10*
Foley's catheter traction 41

hemostatic agents 15, *16*
hemostatic generators 7

insufflator 7
IVC thrombectomy 8, 12

Jackson-Pratt drain 16, *17*

kidney excision completion
    laparoscopic radical nephrectomy 67, *67*
    laparoscopic radical nephroureterectomy
       84, *84*
Kocherization of the duodenum *57*, *75*, *95*, *174*

laparoscopic partial nephresctomy
    access 89–90, *89–91*
    adhesiolysis 91, *92*, *93*
    adrenal gland separation 101
    colon mobilization *93*, 93–94, *94*
    drain insertion 108
    gonadal vessels 96–97, *96–97*
    in left side 95, *96*
    liver retraction 91, *92*, *93*
    operation room setup 91, *92*
    pedicle 98–101
    pedicle clamping 102–103, *102–103*

port insertion 90, *91*
position 89, *89*
posteromedial dissection 97–98, *97–98*
psoas muscle 96–97, *96–97*
renal reconstruction 105–108, *105–108*
in right side 94, *94*, *95*
specimen retrieval 108
surgeon positions 91, *92*
tumor dissection 101–102
tumor resection 103–104, *103–104*
ureter 96–97, *96–97*
wound closure 108
laparoscopic radical cystoprostatectomy
    bladder dropping 126–127, *127–128*
    bladder pedicle control 131–132, *131–132*
    defatting prostate 128, *128*
    division of DVC 133–134, *133–135*
    dorsal vascular complex ligation
       130–131, *130–131*
    dropping bladder 126–127, *127–128*
    endopelvic fascia 128, *128*
    nerve sparing 132–133, *132–133*
    opening endopelvic fascia 129–130,
       129–130
    operating room setup 120, *121*
    port insertion 119–120, *120*
    position 119, *119*
    posterior dissection 124–125, *125,126*
    prostate pedicle 132–133, *132–133*
    Retzius space dissection 126–127, *127–128*
    surgeon positions 120, *121*
    transposition of left ureter to right side 135
    ureteric dissection 121–124, *121–124*
    urethra 133–134, *133–135*
laparoscopic radical nephrectomy
    access 51–52, *52*
    adhesiolysis 53, *54–55*
    adrenalectomy 66
    adrenal gland preservation 65–66, *66*
    colon mobilization 55–56, *55–56*
    drain 67, *67*
    gonadal vessels 58–59, *59–60*
    kidney excision completion 67, *67*
    liver retraction 53, *54–55*
    operating room setup 53, *54*
    pedicle 61–65, *61–65*
    port insertion 52–53, *53*
    position 51, *51*
    posteromedial dissection 60, *60*
    psoas muscle 58–59, *59–60*
    in right side 56–57, *56–57*
    specimen retrieval 67, *67*
    surgeon positions 53, *54*
    upper pole dissection 65–66, *66*
    ureter vessels 58–59, *59–60*
    wound closure 67, *67*

laparoscopic radical nephroureterectomy
    access 69–70, *70*
    additional port insertion 84
    adhesiolysis 71, *72, 73*
    adrenalectomy 84
    adrenal gland preservation 82–83, *82–83*
    bladder cuff excision 85–87, *85–87*
    colon mobilization 73–74, *73–74*
    distal ureteric dissection 85–87, *85–87*
    drains 87
    gonadal vessels *76–77,* 76–78
    kidney excision completion 84, *84*
    liver retraction 71, *72, 73*
    operating room setup 71, *72*
    port insertion 70–71, *71*
    position 69, *69*
    posteromedial dissection 78–82, *78–82*
    psoas muscle *76–77,* 76–78
    specimen retrieval 87
    surgeon positions 71, *72*
    upper pole dissection 82–83, *82–83*
    ureter *76–77,* 76–78
    ureteral mobilization 84, *85*
    wound closure 87
laparoscopic radical prostatectomy
    adhesiolysis 31, *31*
    anterior reconstruction 48, *48*
    bladder neck dissection 39–41, *39–41*
    drain extraction 49
    DVC division 44–45, *45*
    DVC ligation 37–38, *37–38*
    hemostasis 45, *46,* 49
    nerve sparing 43, *43*
    opening endopelvic fascia 35–36, *35–37*
    operating room setup 30, *30*
    port insertion 29–30, *29–30*
    position 29, *29*
    posterior reconstruction 45, *46*
    prostate and endopelvic fascia 34–35, *34–35*
    Retzius space 31–33, *31–34*
    specimen extraction 49
    surgeon positions 30, *30*
    urethral division 44–45, *45*
    vasa and seminal vesicles 41–43, *41–43*
    vesico-urethral anastomosis 46–48, *47–48*
    wound closure 49
laparoscopic Satinsky clamp 12
ligaments
    coronary 56–57, 74, 94, *95,* 173
    hepatorenal 56–57, 74, 94, *95,* 173, *174*
    linorenal *58, 75, 76, 96, 174*
liver retraction 53, *54–55*
lumbar vein 62, *62,* 79, *80,* 99, 100, 114, 177, *178,* 193

Maryland grasper 8, 31, *66, 83, 126*

needle drivers 11, *11*
nerve sparing 43, 44, 125, 132–133, *134,* 160, 161–162
neurovascular bundle (NVB) 41, 44, *45, 46, 131,* 132, 135, 159, 161, *161, 162, 164*

operating room setup
    laparoscopic radical cystoprostatectomy 120, *121*
    laparoscopic radical nephrectomy 53, *54*
    laparoscopic radical nephroureterectomy 71, *72*
    laparoscopic radical prostatectomy 30, *30*
    monitor height 5, *5*
    optimal patient position 3
    patient morbidities 3
    prevent position-related injury 3, *3*
    retroperitoneal laparoscopic nephrectomy 112, *112*
    robotic partial nephrectomy 171, *171*
    robotic radical prostatectomy 151, *151*
    safe patient position 3
    surgeon positions 4, *4*
    surgical complications 3
optiview trocar 21, 29, 52, *52,* 70, 90, 120, 149, 170

pedicle
    laparoscopic partial nephrectomy 98–101
    retroperitoneal laparoscopic nephrectomy 114–115, *114–116*
    robotic partial nephrectomy *177,* 177–178, *179*
pedicle clamping
    laparoscopic partial nephrectomy 102–103, *102–103*
    retroperitoneal robotic partial nephrectomy *195,* 195–196
    robotic partial nephrectomy 180–181, *181*
pneumoperitoneum 22, 29, 52, 70, 90, 111, 120, 143, 149, 170, 189
port configuration 24–25, *24–25*
port insertion
    laparoscopic partial nephrectomy 90, *91*
    laparoscopic radical nephrectomy 52–53, *53*
    laparoscopic radical nephroureterectomy 70–71, *71*
    laparoscopic radical prostatectomy 29–30, *29–30*
    robotic radical prostatectomy 149–150, *150*
port site closure 25, *25*
position
    laparoscopic partial nephrectomy 89, *89*
    laparoscopic radical cystoprostatectomy 119, *119*
    laparoscopic radical nephrectomy 51, *51*

position (*cont.*)
   laparoscopic radical nephroureterectomy 69, *69*
   laparoscopic radical prostatectomy 29, *29*
   operating room setup 3
   retroperitoneal laparoscopic nephrectomy 109, *109*
   retroperitoneal robotic partial nephrectomy 187, *188*
   robotic partial nephrectomy 169, *169*
   robotic radical prostatectomy 149, *149*
posterior bladder neck reconstruction 40, *40*, 41, 45, 157, *158*, 164, *165*, *166*
posteromedial dissection
   laparoscopic partial nephrectomy 97–98, *97–98*
   laparoscopic radical nephroureterectomy 78–82, *78–82*
   robotic partial nephrectomy *176*, 176–177, *177*
prostatic pedicle, robotic radical prostatectomy 158–161, *159–161*

radical nephrectomy 8
renal hilum 52, 57, 74, 90, 94, *114*, 173
renal pedicle, dissection/clip ligation 108, 185, 194, 200
renorrhaphy 15, *16*, 102, 103, 106, *106*, 107, *107*, 108, 181, 185, *185*, 199, *199*, 200
retractors 10, *10*
retroperitoneal laparoscopic nephrectomy
   access 109–111, *110–111*
   adrenal gland preservation 117, *117*
   drain insertion 117
   first trocar insertion 109–111, *110–111*
   Gerota's fascia dissection 112–114, *113–114*
   kidney dissection completion 116–117, *116–117*
   ligation of ureter 116–117, *116–117*
   operating room setup 112, *112*
   other trocar insertions *111*, 111–112
   pedicle 114–115, *114–116*
   position 109, *109*
   psoas muscle dissection 112–114, *113–114*
   specimen retrieval 117
   surgeon positions 112, *112*
   upper pole dissection 117, *117*
   wound closure 117
retroperitoneal robotic partial nephrectomy
   access 187, *189*, 189–190
   assisting surgeon 191, *191*
   drain insertion 200
   first trocar insertion 187, *189*, 189–190
   Gerota's fascia dissection 191–192, *192*
   hilar dissection *193*, 193–194, *194*
   pedicle clamping *195*, 195–196

position 187, *188*
renal reconstruction 197–200, *197–200*
robotic trocars insertion 190, *190*
specimen retrieval 200
the robotic instruments 191, *191*
tumor dissection 194
tumor resection *196*, 196–197, *197*
wound closure 200
Retzius space 31–33, *31–34*
   dissection 126–127, *127–128*
   entering 151–153, *152–154*
right-angled dissector 8
robotic partial nephrectomy
   access 169–170, *170*, *171*
   adhesiolysis 171–172, *172*
   adrenal gland 180
   assisting surgeons 171, *171*
   colon mobilization 172–173, *173*
   docking of robot 170, *171*
   drain insertion 186, *186*
   first port insertion 170
   gonadal vessels 175, *175*
   in left side 173, *174*, 175
   liver retraction 171–172, *172*
   operating room setup 171, *171*
   pedicle clamping 180–181, *181*
   position 169, *169*
   posteromedial dissection *176*, 176–177, *177*
   psoas muscle 175, *175*
   renal reconstruction 183–186, *183–186*
   robotic four arm instruments 170
   robotic trocar insertion 170, *171*
   specimen retrieval 186, *186*
   the pedicle *177*, 177–178, *179*
   tumor dissection 180, *180*
   tumor resection 181–183, *182–183*
   ureter 175, *175*
   wound closure 186, *186*
robotic radical prostatectomy
   adhesiolysis 151, *152*
   anterior reconstruction 167, *168*
   assistant surgeon positions 151, *151*
   bladder neck dissection 156–158, *157–158*
   defatting prostate 155–156, *155–156*
   dorsal vascular complex 156
   drain 168
   dropping bladder 151–154
   DVC suturing 163–164
   DVC transection *162*, 162–163
   endopelvic fascia 155–156, *155–156*
   entering Retzius space 151–153, *152–154*
   hemostasis 163–164, 168
   nerve sparing 161–162, *161–162*
   operating room setup 151, *151*
   port insertion 149–150, *150*
   position 149, *149*

posterior reconstruction 164, *165*
prostatic pedicle 158–161, *159–161*
seminal vesicles 158–161, *159–161*
specimen extraction 168
urethral division *162,* 162–163
vas deference 158–161, *159–161*
vesicourethral anastomosis 165–167, *165–167*
wound closure 168
Rocco stitch 45–46, 164–165

scissors 13
Secteroization 126
sling stitch 48, *168*
specimen retrieval approaches 16, *16*
    laparoscopic partial nephrectomy 108
    laparoscopic radical nephrectomy 67, *67*
    laparoscopic radical nephroureterectomy 87
    retroperitoneal laparoscopic nephrectomy 117
    retroperitoneal robotic partial nephrectomy 200
    robotic partial nephrectomy 186, *186*
S-shape retractors 10, *10*
staplers 14–15, *15*
Studer orthotopic ileal neobladder 137–145
suction-irrigation functions 8, *9*
surgeon positions
    laparoscopic partial nephrectomy 91, *92*
    laparoscopic radical cystoprostatectomy 120, *121*
    laparoscopic radical nephrectomy 53, *54*
    laparoscopic radical nephroureterectomy 71, *72*
    laparoscopic radical prostatectomy 30, *30*
    operating room setup 4, *4*
    retroperitoneal laparoscopic nephrectomy 112, *112*
    surgeon posture 4, *4*
surgeon posture
    monitor height 5, *5*
    optimal patient position 3
    patient morbidities 3
    prevent position-related injury 3, *3*
    safe patient position 3
    surgeon positions 4, *4*
    surgical complications 3
surgical instruments and machines
    Bulldog vascular clamps 12, *13*
    camera (laparoscope) 8
    clips and clip applicators *13,* 13–14, *14*
    da Vinci Xi robotic cart 7, 21
    drains 16, *17*
    energy devices 7
    fan retractor 10, *10*
    hemostatic agents 15, *16*

    hemostatic generators 7
    insufflator 7
    Jackson-Pratt drain 16, *17*
    needle drivers 11, *11*
    retractors 10, *10*
    scissors 13
    specimen retrieval 16, *16*
    S-shape retractors 10, *10*
    staplers 14–15, *15*
    suction-irrigation functions 8, *9*
    surgical sterile table 8
    sutures 11
    suturing maneuver 11–12, *12*
    ultrasound probe 8
surgical sterile table 8
sutures 11
suturing maneuver 11–12, *12*

TachoSil roll 15, *16,* 107, 185, *185,* 199, *199*
Trendelenburg position 29, *29*
triangulation principle, port placement 70, *71*
trocar 21, *21,* 22
    insertions 22–23, *22–23*

ultrasonic shears 7, 39, *39,* 62, *100,* 100, 121, *124,* 132
ultrasound probe 8
urinary diversion, step-by-step surgery
    ileal segment isolation 137–138, *138*
    intestinal continuity restoration 139, *139*
    neobladder reconstruction 140–141, *140–141*
    uretero-ileal anastomosis 141, *142,* 143
    urethra-neobladder anastomosis 143–145, *143–145*

veress needle 7, 8, *19,* 19–20, *20,* 29, 30, 51, 52, 69, 70, 71, 89, 90, 119, 120, 150, *170,* 170
vesicourethral anastamosis 11, 33, 39, 45, *47, 48,* 153, 157, 164, 165–167

wound closure
    laparoscopic partial nephrectomy 108
    laparoscopic radical cystoprostatectomy 135, *136*
    laparoscopic radical nephrectomy 67, *67*
    laparoscopic radical nephroureterectomy 87
    laparoscopic radical prostatectomy 49
    retroperitoneal laparoscopic nephrectomy 117
    retroperitoneal robotic partial nephrectomy 200
    robotic partial nephrectomy 186, *186*
    robotic radical prostatectomy 168

Index

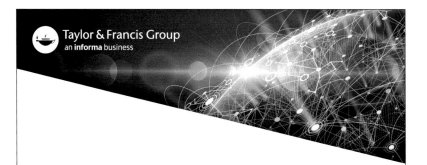